Clinical Handbook

D1743275

ORAL

Medicine &

Pathology

from A-Z

Henning Lehmann Bastian

Henning Lehmann Bastian

Clinical Handbook

ORAL Medicine & Pathology from A-Z

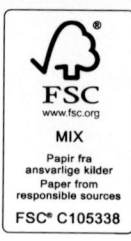

© 2015 Henning Lehmann Bastian
Publisher: BoD - Copenhagen, Denmark
Production: BoD - Norderstedt, Germany

ISBN 978-87-7145-474-1

Foreword

The book is intended as a clinical guide for the practising dentist, but dentistry students, practitioners and ear, nose and throat doctors will also be able to make use of the book as a reference. The book has included in the form of a lexicon only the most common conditions in Oral Medicine and Pathology. If you are interested and would like to go deeper into each topic, you are recommended to visit the major electronic search engines such as PubMed and Grateful Med.

At the back of the book there is a so-called "diagnostic tree" by which on the basis of symptoms and clinical signs it is possible to achieve an approximate diagnosis in the particular case in oral medicine. In addition, there is also a text on electronic search for the benefit of students.

Constructive criticism and suggestions for improvement are welcome. Also interesting clinical profiles. Contact: hlb@os.dk.

Copenhagen 1/12-2014

Henning Lehmann Bastian

About the Author

Henning Lehmann Bastian is a trained dentist with further training as a specialist in oral- and maxillofacial surgery. He was for many years head of the Department of oral- and maxillofacial surgery at Odense University and a lecturer at the Aarhus School of Dentistry in the subject Oral Medicine and Pathology. He has for many years been an external examiner in the subject Oral surgery, medicine and pathology at the two dental schools in Denmark. He is the specialist editor of the website www.tandogmund.dk. He also worked as a forensic odontologist in cooperation with the Forensic Medicine Institute, Odense University from 1974-2013.

The author has been a leader in the study of implants in Denmark and in 1998 started up the Danish section of the ITI of which he was Chairman until 2008. Since 2009, he has been a member of the "international expert committee" for Camlog.

He has previously published the books "Teeth leave traces", "Oral Medicine" and the children's books "Tandsylvania" and "Tandsylvania Zoo". In addition, he has written a chapter in the book "Wounds" and in the online version of "General practice" for practitioners. He has also written more than a hundred professional articles, mainly in Danish, but also in foreign, journals.

Content

1. Abrasio dentium

Definition: Wear of enamel/dentin caused otherwise than by tooth contact.

Aetiology: Abrasion has a variable pattern, depending on the cause of the wear. Typically toothbrush damage at the transition between enamel and dentine Fig.1.1. Abrasion is also seen on the incisal edge e.g. after use of the teeth to hold pins, wire, nails etc.. There is also the well-known abrasion from the mouthpiece in habitual pipe smokers Fig.1.2. Sustained use of toothpicks may result in atypical approximal wear.

Symptoms: Since abrasion develops over a long time there is seldom dentine hypersensitivity, due to the formation of secondary dentine.

Clinical features: It is easy to recognise the damage by ordinary visual examination. Fig.1.3.

Diagnosis: The diagnosis is performed clinically

Treatment: The treatment will be the correction of the unfortunate dental care habits and conservative dentistry, possibly reconstruction.

Differential diagnosis: Erosions.

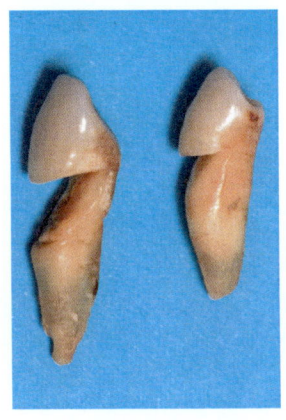

Fig. 1.1.

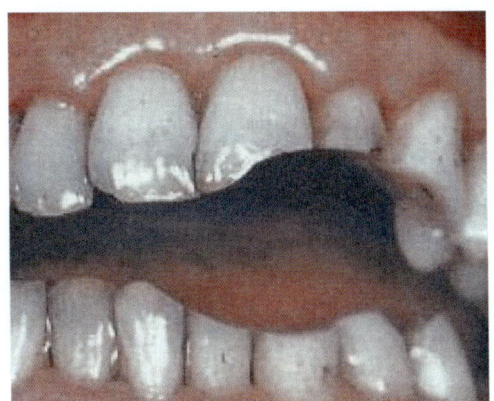

Fig. 1.2.

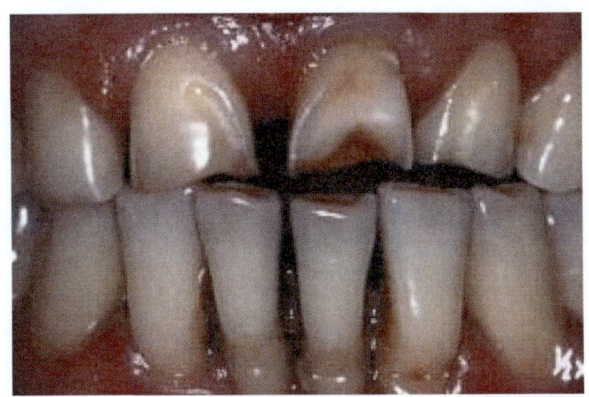

Fig. 1.3.

2. Abscessus parodontalis

Definition: An abscess has occurred in an existing periodontal pocket.

Aetiology: The abscess occurs when the degradation of the bone around a tooth has resulted in the formation of a deep periodontal pocket, and the secretion of pus from it is blocked. Through the closure of the pocket pus accumulates and an abscess forms. The condition can also result from changes in the bacterial flora in the pocket, an impaired immune system or a combination of these factors. Most frequently seen in adults. In children, it can be seen in cases of cutting of teeth.

Symptoms: Strong throbbing pain, aggravated by chewing and pressure on the tooth. Causes bad breath. In acute cases there is swelling and tenderness of proximal lymph nodes and fever. The responsible tooth can be easily identified and in addition to the pain the tooth is often loose to a greater or lesser degree.

Clinical features: Gums are erythematous and oedematous with a raised red surface. By probing into the pocket the pus can be expressed. Fig.2.1.

Diagnosis: The diagnosis can be performed clinical, radiological and possibly by swab.

Treatment: The acute treatment includes incision, drainage and antibiotic therapy. The further treatment may take the form of extraction, or parodontal surgical intervention in order to preserve the tooth.

Differential diagnosis: Pyogenic granuloma. Apical abscess. Gingiva cyst.

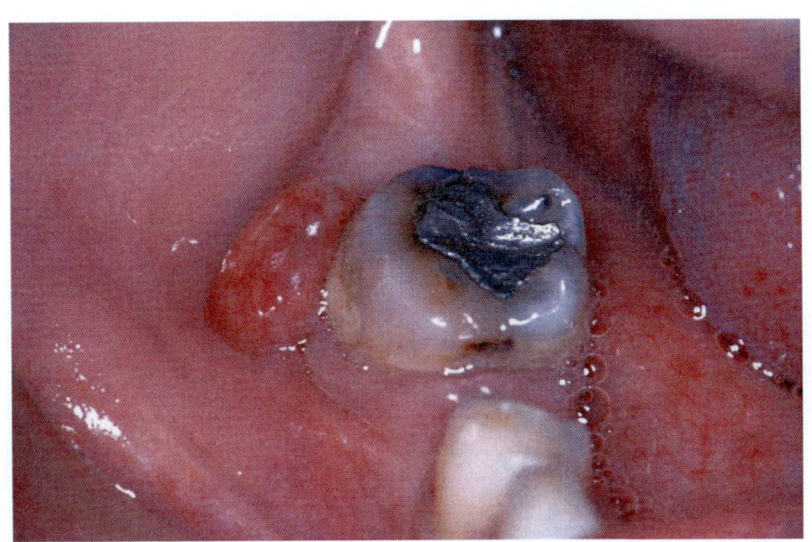

Fig. 2.1.

3. Abscessus periapikalis

Definition: An abscess has occurred in the root tip of an avital tooth.

Aetiology: Pulp necrosis. The chronic periapical process can develop into a parulis or radicular cyst.

Symptoms: The chronic form is asymptomatic. The acute form is particularly characterized by pain.

Clinical features: Submucosal swelling and possibly fluctuation produces a tooth abscess, **parulis** Fig.3.1. The vast majority of dental abscesses perforate the cheek. In the upper jaw they can also perforate the palate Fig.3.2. In the molars in the lower jaw, in rare cases, the development of a gravity abscess can be seen with the risk of airway obstruction, requiring hospitalisation. The **unilateral maxillary sinusitis** almost always comes from a tooth root. If a patient develops an abscess **at the lower pole of the tonsil** it may come from the wisdom tooth on the same side. In rare cases **osteomyelitis** may develop, Fig.3.3.

Diagnosis: Diagnosis is performed on the clinical, radiological image and possibly swab.

Treatment: The tooth abscess incised and drainage maintained for a few days. There is trepanning of the tooth pulp and a drain is created. Similarly antibiotic therapy is commenced, often 2-drug therapy. Root canal treatment or removal of the tooth.

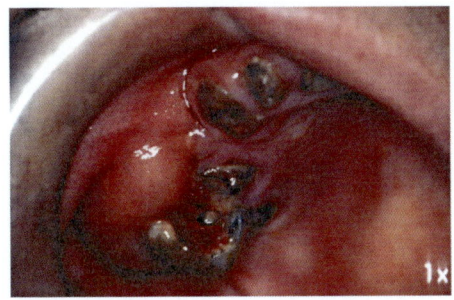

Fig. 3.1.

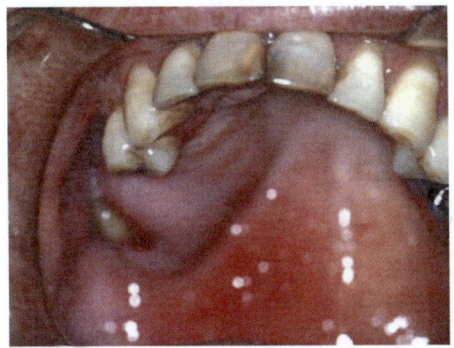

Fig. 3.2.

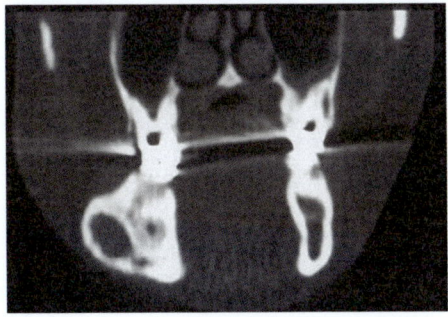

Fig. 3.3.

4. Acromegalia

Definition: Extra growth of the face, hands and feet after epiphyseal closure.

Aetiology: Overproduction of growth hormone, most often due to a pituitary adenoma.

Symptoms: Headache, hypertension, heart disease, hyper-hidrosis, arthritis and peripheral neuropathy. Typically, an enlargement of the head - the patient has to wear a larger hat. The nose, lips, zygomatic arch and eyebrows also grow. Intraorally that is growth of the maxilla and especially mandible with progenism as a result. Spreading of the teeth, often exacerbated by the pressure from the enlarged tongue.

Clinical features: The clinical features will be characterised by the above symptoms. A prognathic mandible and spreading is often an early sign. Fig.4.1 shows a relatively young man who has received implants before the disease began. It is seen how the jaw has grown but the ancylosed implants have not followed Fig.4.2. On the X-ray image in Fig.4.3 implants can be seen to "hang" high in the bone.

Diagnosis: X-ray and blood tests will provide the answer.

Treatment: A curative therapy is the removal of the adenoma or rays. The oral problems can be treated by a orthognate surgical intervention, but it is necessary ensure that the growth is finished.

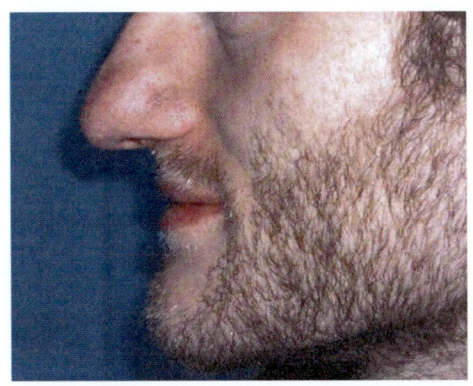

Fig. 4.1.

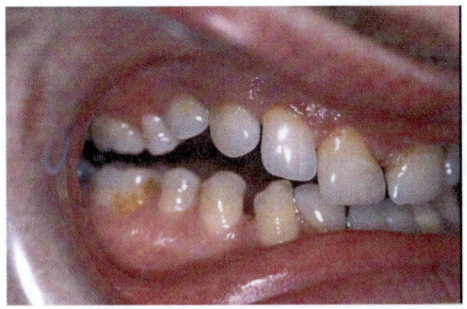

Fig. 4.2.

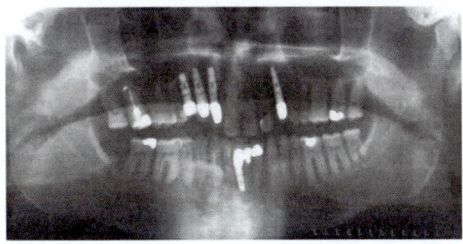

Fig. 4.3.

5. Actinomycosis cervico-facialis

Definition: A chronic granulomatous infection.

Aetiology: The infection is caused by actinomyces israelii. Often you will find accompanying flora with streptococci or staphylococci. Actinomyces is found occasionally in the saliva.

Symptoms: Actinomycose seldom causes pain, but often trismus. It presents itself as a board hard, red or purple swelling on the skin. In the typical case there are multiple fistulas with small yellow sulphur grains and small abscesses.

Clinical features: The infection is seen as a chronic, slowly growing process Fig.5.1. Actinomycose should be considered if the infection with extraoral swelling does not respond within two weeks to conventional treatment with antibiotics and targeted therapy Fig.5.2. The number of cases peaks in May and November.

Diagnosis: Small abscesses and clearance of sulphur granules in the pus from an abscess is diagnostic of Actinomycose. Fig.5.3 shows the yellow sulphur granules in the pus. The diagnosis is performed by anaerobic culture of the material from an abscess or biopsy. Many prefer a fine needle aspirate.

Treatment: Drainage is often disappointing. Metronidazole for 10 days, for example 500 mg. 3 times/day and Penicillin for 4-6 weeks. Targeted therapy.

Differential diagnosis: Classic absces.

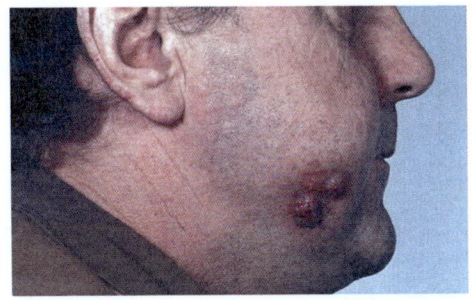

Fig. 5.1.

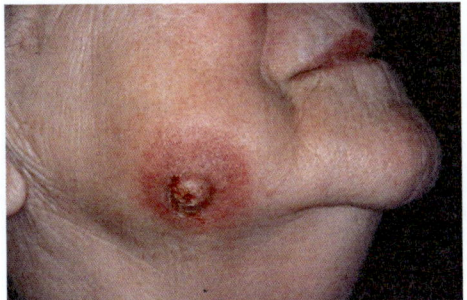

Fig. 5.2.

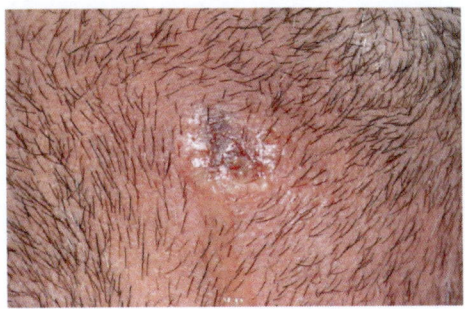

Fig. 5.3.

23

6. Acute necrotizing gingivitis

Definition: Specific gingival infectious disease in younger people.

Aetiology: This is an anaerobic infection mainly with fusobacteria and spirochetes. The prevalence in the general population today is less than 0.1%.However, with HIV infection the disease has undergone a "renaissance".

Symptoms: The patient has pronounced halitosis, and there is significant pain. Food intake may not be possible because of the pain and bleeding from the gingiva.

Clinical features: The destruction of the periodontal tissues starts in typical cases on top of the gingival papillae Fig.6.1. After a period of pronounced inflammatory changes, the tissue becomes necrotic Fig.6.2. There are punched, crater-like necroses covered with a greyish pseudomembrane.

Diagnosis: Performed on the basis of the clinical profile.

Treatment: General antibiotic treatment in particular with metronidazole. Intraoral topical treatment with chlorhexidine or 1% hydrogen peroxide as a flush or spray. In addition, scaling and instruction in oral hygiene. Currently one should recommend HIV testing.

Differential diagnosis: Herpetic gingivostomatitis. Erythema multiforme. Agranulocytosis. Leukaemia.

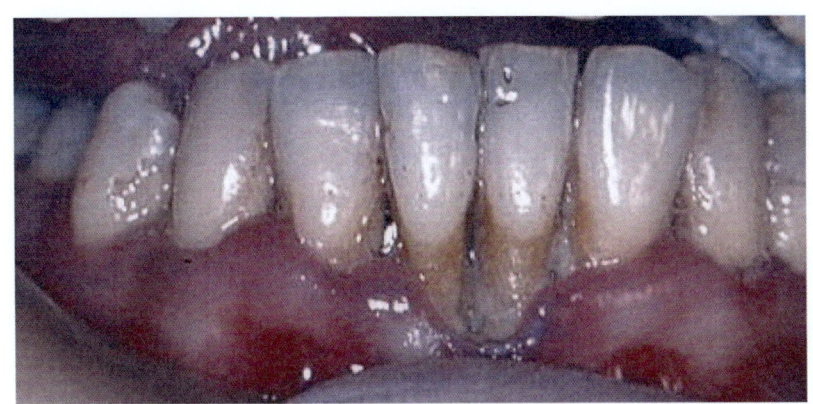

Fig. 6.1.

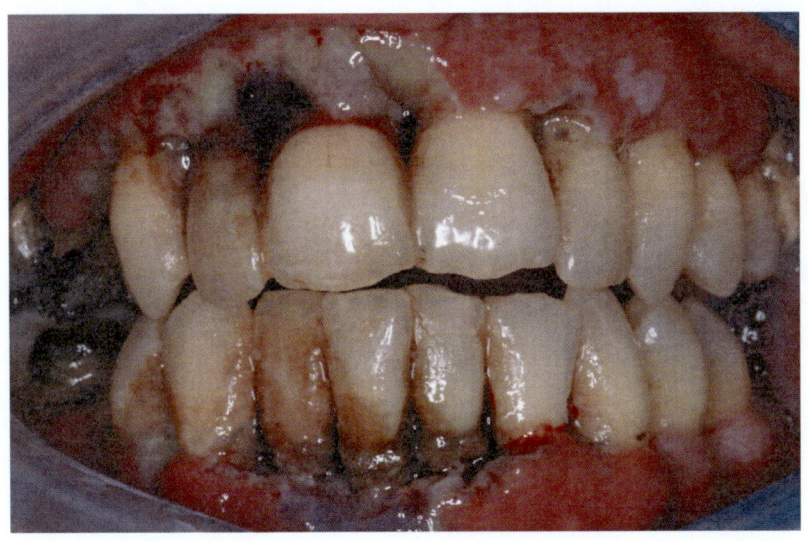

Fig. 6.2.

7. Adenoma pleomorphicum

Definition: A benign saliva gland tumour.

Aetiology: unknown

Symptoms: painless, slow-growing swelling.

Clinical features: The tumour is also called mixed tumour and is the most common saliva gland tumour, mostly in gl.parotis. The patient has often had a tumour long before she/he comes for treatment. The tumour occurs in all age groups but is most common between 30 and 50 years. It occurs more often in women. Intraorally the tumour is seen most frequently in the palate beyond the molars. In clinical terms a vaulted mass with a smooth surface is seen, Fig.7.1 and Fig.7.2. Fig.7.3. shows an atypical case in the cheek.

Diagnosis: A fine needle biopsy can be taken for histological examination.

Treatment: The adenoma is removed by surgical excision. The tumour must be removed completely up to bone contact, including the periosteum and overlying mucous membrane. The prognosis is good and there is little tendency to relapse, but in 5% of cases there is a risk of malignant transformation. Treatment is a specialist task.

Differential diagnosis: Adenocystic carcinoma, Lymphoma.

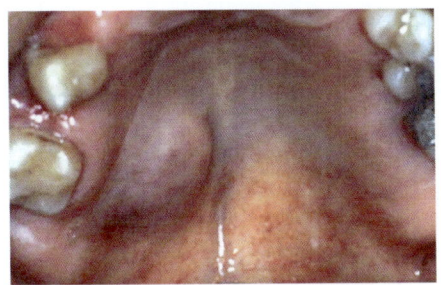

Fig. 7.1.

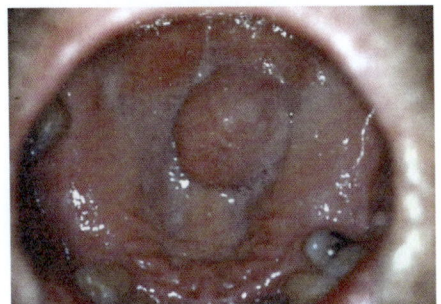

Fig. 7.2.

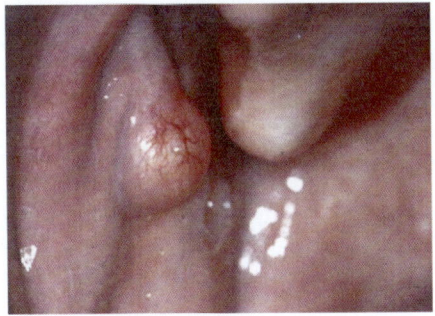

Fig. 7.3.

8. AIDS and HIV

Definition: Infection by the HIV virus.

Aetiology: The cause is an immunodeficiency caused by the HIV virus.

Symptoms: Due to the weakened immunity there are many infections, viruses, fungi Fig.8.1 and bacteria Fig.8.2. Also, carcinomas, lymphomas and non-Hodgkins lymphomas, Kaposi sarcoma and on the tongue side rim the familiar Hairy Leukoplakia Fig.8.3 which resembles a snail trail.

Clinical features: The oral clinical manifestations are totally dependent on the progression of the disease.

Diagnosis: Can be performed on a blood sample.

Treatment: Treatment is a specialist task. The dentist may treat the oral diseases as they occur.

Differential diagnosis: Other immunodeficiency disease.

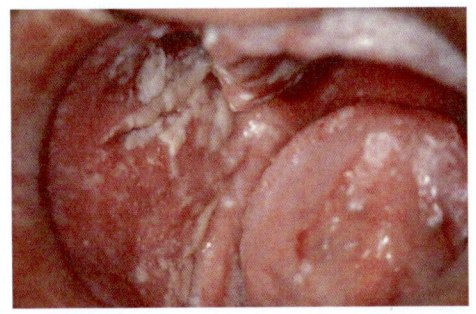

Fig. 8.1.

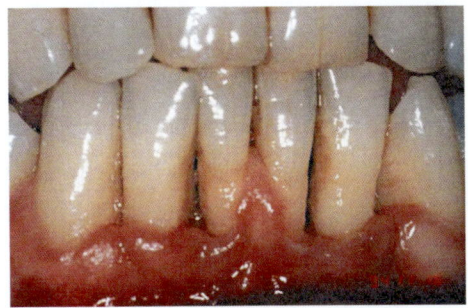

Fig. 8.2.

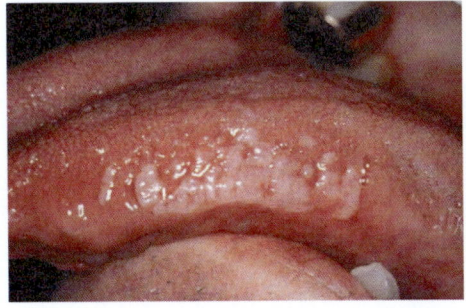

Fig. 8.3.

9. Amalgam tattoo

Definition: Blue or blue-black discoloration of the mucous membrane

Aetiology: Amalgam left in the mucous membrane

Symptoms: None

Clinical features: A blue/blue-black discoloration of the gingiva or the nearest mucosa Fig.9.1. Fig.9.2 shows the case of prevalent amalgam discoloration.

Diagnosis: The diagnosis can only be performed properly by taking a biopsy. In the case described, a biopsy is taken to exclude malignant melanoma.

Treatment: None or surgical removal.

Differential diagnosis: Melanoma.

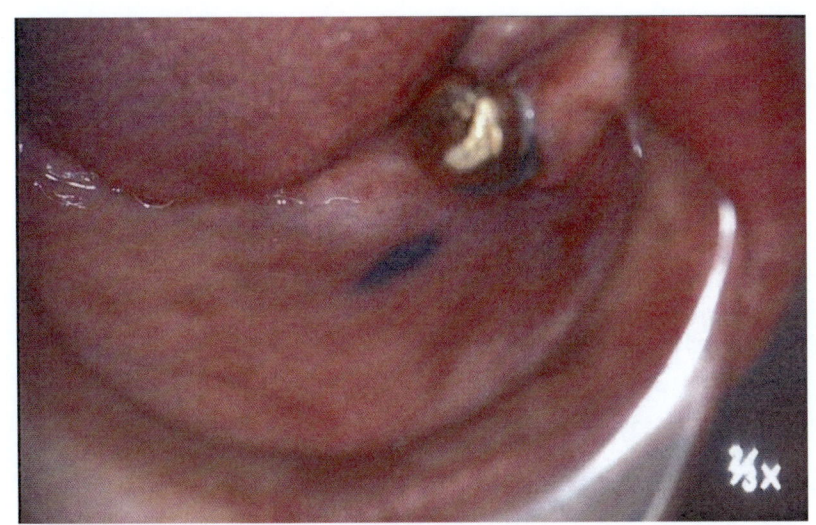

Fig. 9.1.

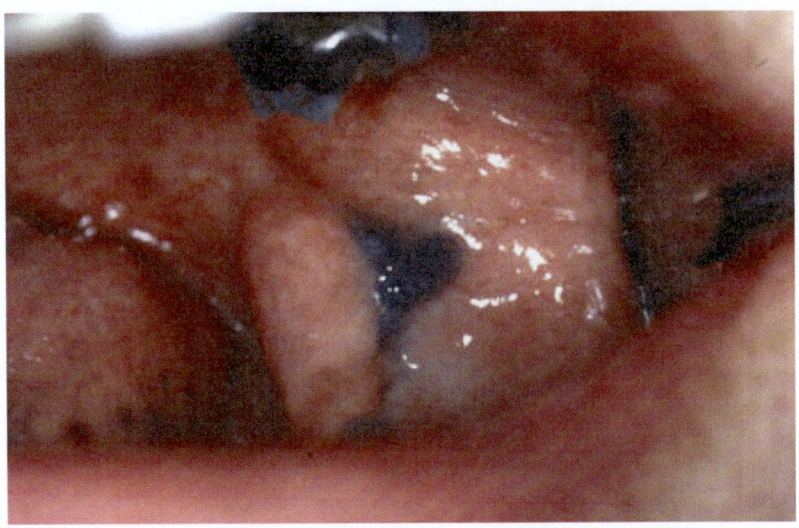

Fig. 9.2.

10. Ambustio

Definition: Burns of the mucous membrane.

Aetiology: Varies, but in children often electrical wiring.

Symptoms: Pain.

Clinical features: There are ulcerations in the lip region or in the mouth and tongue. Fig.10.1 shows a burn on the upper lip after a cigarette was inserted with the burning end first.

Diagnosis: The diagnosis is performed on the basis of a thorough medical history.

Treatment: Soothing creams such as a mixture of lidocaine and chlorohexidine. Healing is often very slow.

Differential diagnosis: In the absence of healing, c.oris must be considered.

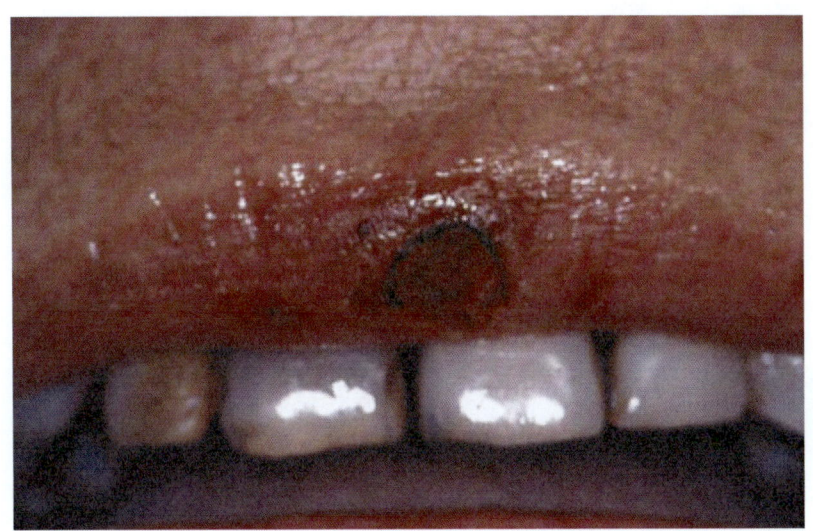

Fig. 10.1.

11. Ameloblastoma

Definition: Odontogenic tumour.

Aetiology: Unknown.

Symptoms: Asymptomatic. Swelling, but rarely pain or paresthesia. Dental migration can be seen. Root resorption is also seen.

Clinical features: Most common in the 30-50 years age group. 85% in the mandible. A large X-ray image such as an OP-recording will reveal a usually quite large clearing with a multilocular or unilocular appearance Fig.11.1, Fig.11.2. A Ct scan, Fig.11.3 shows how the tumour is locally aggressive.

Diagnosis: The diagnosis can only be precisely histological. There are several sub-groups.

Treatment: Specialist task. The current consensus is that the treatment is local resection. There is a great tendency to relapse after the multilocular type. The unilocular type shows recurrence in 10-20% of cases. There can be malignant transformation of the ameloblastoma and the development of a carcinoma in the ameloblastoma has been observed.

Differential diagnosis: Keratocyst.

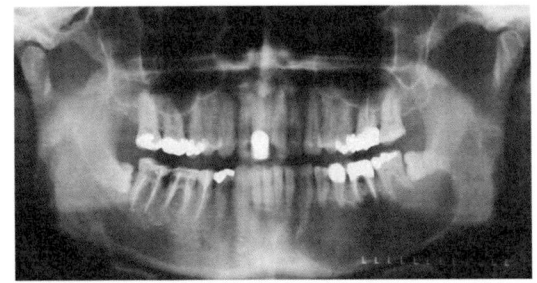

Fig. 11.1.

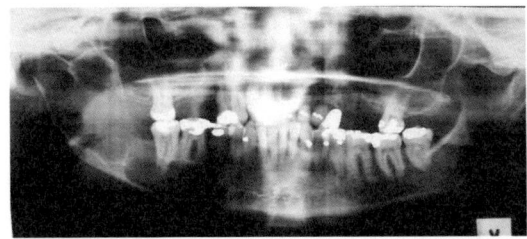

Fig. 11.2.

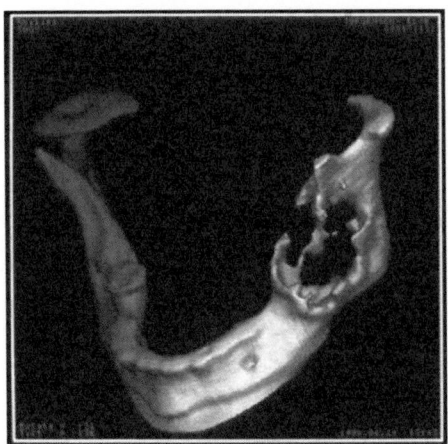

Fig. 11.3.

12. Amelogenesis imperfecta

Definition: Congenital abnormality of the tooth enamel.

Aetiology: Unknown.

Symptoms: The tooth enamel shell and dentine are exposed. Very sensitive teeth. Cosmetically compromising.

Clinical features: There are 3 types: the hypomineralised, Fig.12.1 and the hypoplastic, Fig.12.2 and Fig.12.3, and the immature type! Seen in 1 out of 16,000 individuals. Occurs both in the primary and permanent dentition. Often worst in the permanent dentition. The three types often occur simultaneously. There is considerable wear, which is why the disorder is associated with significant functional, cosmetic and therapeutic problems.

Diagnosis: The diagnosis can be performed on a thorough medical history, clinical findings and histology.

Treatment: The disorder causes major medical problems. Intensive prophylaxis. Will often end up with a total dental reconstruction.

Differential diagnosis: Dental fluorosis. Dentinogenesis imperfecta. Systematic external enamel hypoplasia.

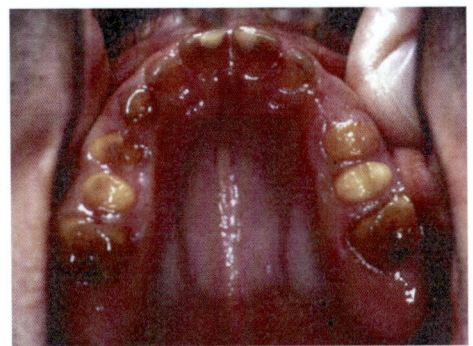

Fig. 12.1.

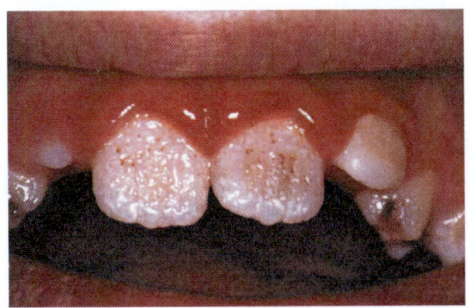

Fig. 12.2.

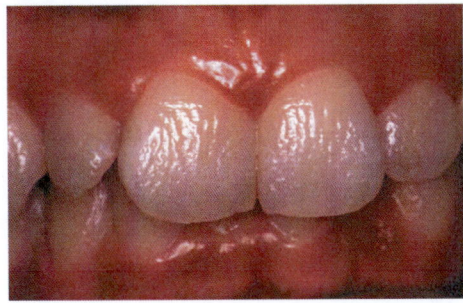

Fig. 12.3.

37

13. Amyloidosis

Definition: Metabolic disorder characterised by extracellular deposition of a proteinaceous substance called amyloid.

Aetiology: Unknown. It is a heterogeneous group of syndromes. The composition of the amyloidfibrilla forms the basis for classification.

Symptoms: Symptoms depend on the anatomical distribution and severity of the amyloid deposits. Altzheimers disease is perhaps the most common form of amyloidosis. It is characterised by gradual progressive dementia.

Clinical features: Varied clinical profile. Fatigue, weight loss, paraesthesia, hoarseness, oedema and hypertension. Intraorally macroglossia, Fig.13.1, multiple red tumours, petechiae, bruising, Fig.13.2, ulcerations and bullae, Fig.13.3, are often seen. There may be saliva gland infiltrations which will cause Xerostomia.

Diagnosis: Performed by a biopsy.

Treatment: Treatment is symptomatic.

Differential diagnosis: Kaposi's sarcoma. Crohn's disease. Macroglossia.

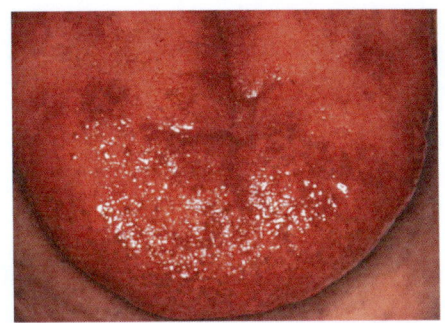

Fig. 13.1.

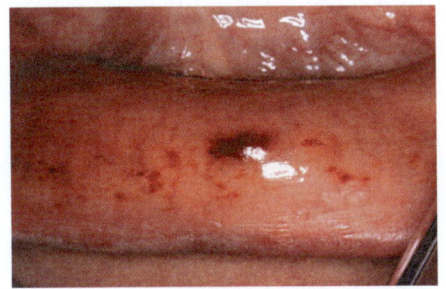

Fig. 13.2.

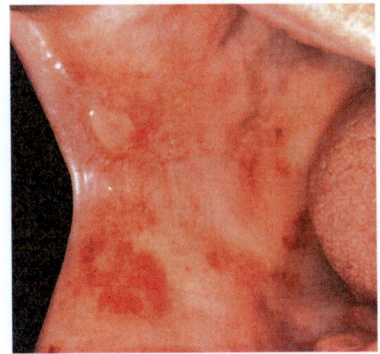

Fig. 13.3.

14. Anaemia perniciosa

Definition: Anaemia due to the absence of Cobalamin B12.

Aetiology: Lack of intrinsic factor in the stomach.

Symptoms: Patients complain of fatigue, headaches, weakness, burning sensation in the tongue, lips or buccal mucous membrane.

Clinical features: Erythema and papilatrophy with lobulation of the upper surface of the tongue. Fig.14.1 are observed. The hair often turns white in a short time and there are paresthesias in tongue, fingers and toes. Also, painful swallowing. Fig.14.2 and Fig.14.3 show the papilla sample before and after the addition of vitamin B.

Diagnosis: Performed from symptoms and a blood sample from the patient's physician.

Treatment: Administration of Vitamin B12

Differential diagnosis: Iron deficiency anaemia. Burning mouth syndrome. Candidiasis oralis.

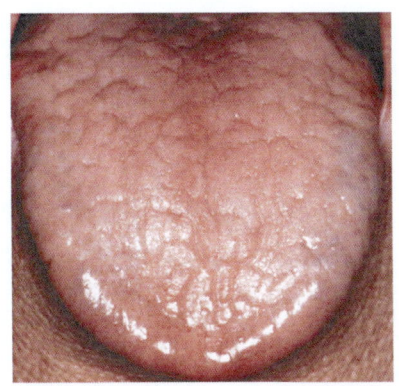

Fig. 14.1.

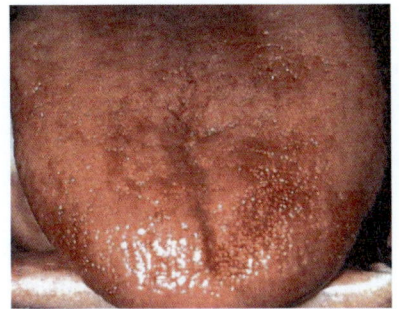

Fig. 14.2.

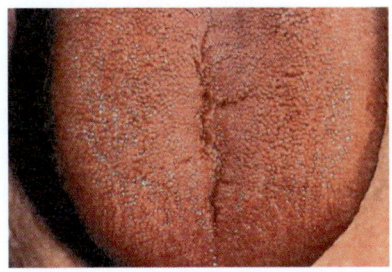

Fig. 14.3.

15. Anaemia sideropenica

Definition: Anaemia due to iron deficiency.

Aetiology: Occurs when iron stores are depleted. Either too small supply of iron or bleeding.

Symptoms: Fatigue and lack of energy. Stinging and burning sensation in the tongue. The nails become soft and concave. Conjuctivae are dry and pale.

Clinical features: Orally there is increasing atrophy of the papillae on the upper surface of the tongue and a generalised atrophy of the mucous membranes, Fig.15.1 and Fig.15.2. Fig.15.3. shows the atrophic buccal mucosa.

Diagnosis: The patient is referred to the doctor for blood test and diagnostics.

Treatment: The cause must be verified. Administration of iron and possibly changing diets. The changes in the tongue will be normalised within 1-2 months.

Differential diagnosis: Candidosis. Anaemia perniciosa.

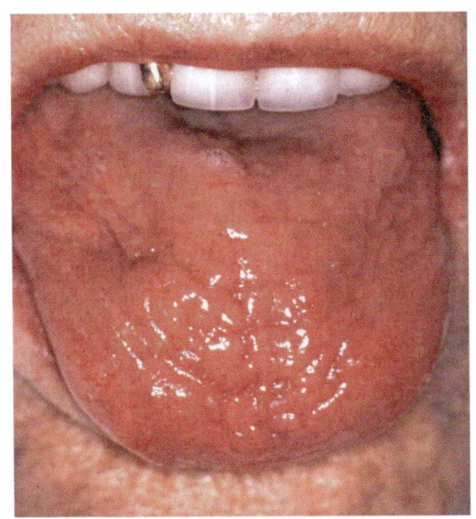

Fig. 15.1.

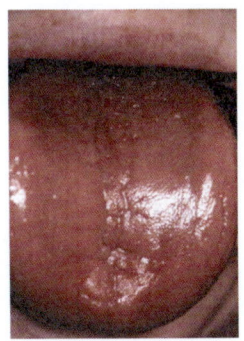

Fig. 15.2.

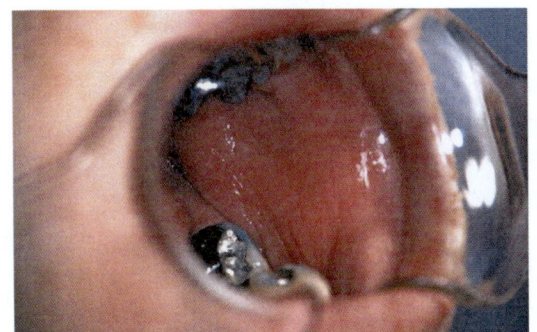

Fig. 15.3.

16. Aneurysmal bone cyst

Definition: Benign intraosseous lesion with blood-filled gaps.

Aetiology: Unknown.

Symptoms: Fast-growing swelling with or without pain.

Clinical features: There is extra oral and intra-oral swelling. Most frequent in the long bones, rare in the jaws. Most often in younger patients, both in the maxilla and mandible. Most frequent in women. X-rays will reveal a unilocular or multilocular, soap bubble type clearing, most commonly in the molar region Fig.16.1. Often the lumen will move up between the teeth roots. Fig.16.2 shows a cutaneous fistula from an infected aneurysmal bone cyst.

Diagnosis: The diagnosis is performed on histological examination.

Treatment: Surgical curettage. The cortex is always extremely thin and there may be excessive bleeding from the lesion. Treatment is a specialist task.

Differential diagnosis: Simple bone cyst. Central giant cell granuloma. Cyst.

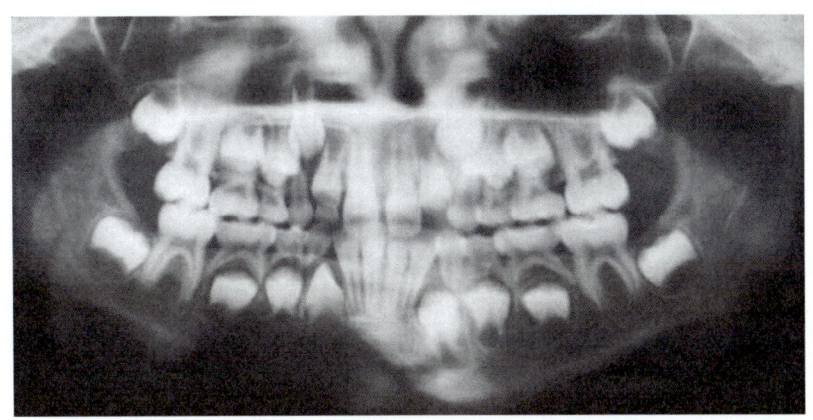

Fig. 16.1.

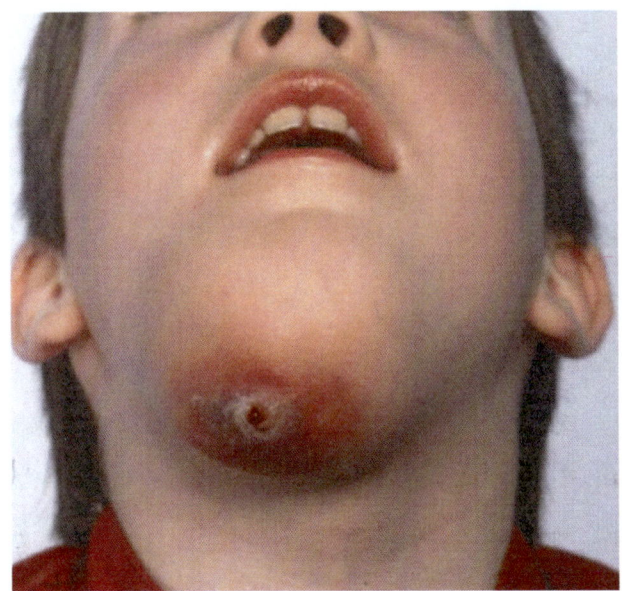

Fig. 16.2.

17. Aphthous stomatitis

Definition: Recurrent ulceration of the oral mucosa. Known by several other names , such as aphthae, stomatitis aphthosa recidivans or blister. Affects 10-30% of the population.

Aetiology: Unknown

Symptoms: Recurrent sores on the oral mucous membrane. The disease starts with itching in the area which subsequently fills with painful ulcerations, which occur in several places and at varying intervals. The pain is worst in the SARC type. Inhibits food intake. There is rarely fever.

Clinical features: Grayish yellow, fibrin coated ulcerations with a red rim (halo) around them. Appearing on non-keratinized mucous membrane frequently in cheeks, lips, tongue, mouth floor and soft palate. Lasts about 8-10 days. Fig.17.1, Fig.17.2 and Fig.17.3. SARC forms scar tissue in the mucous membrane after healing (s.280).

Diagnosis: The histological profile is uncharacteristic. The diagnosis is performed clinically.

Treatment: None or steroid (e.g. Synalar).

Differential diagnosis: Herpetic gingivostomatitis. Varicella. SARC.

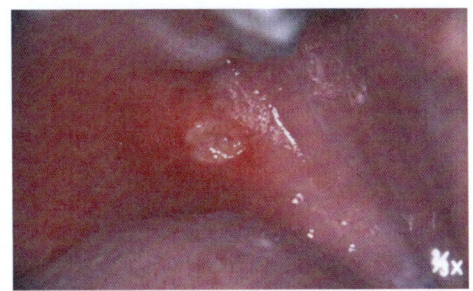

Fig. 17.1.

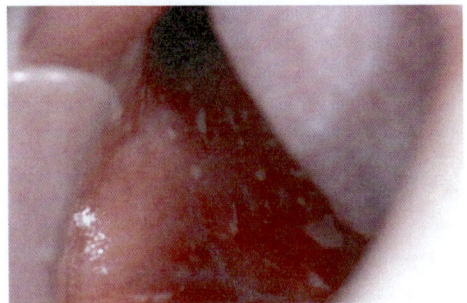

Fig. 17.2.

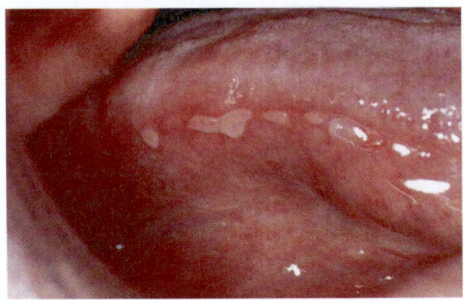

Fig. 17.3.

18. Aplasia dentis

Definition: Missing tooth germ. Also called hypodontia, agenesis and with total lack of dental germ: Anodontia.

Aetiology: Genetic defect, which is often hereditary.

Symptoms: None, but functional and cosmetic deficit.

Clinical features: Appears only after normal tooth eruption, spaces between the teeth. Occurs in 3-10% of a year. The most frequently missing tooth is the second premolar, followed by the lateral incisor in the upper jaw. Fig.18.1, Fig.18.2 and Fig.18.3.

Diagnosis: Missing tooth germ. Can be verified on a radiograph.

Treatment: Orthodontics or implantological reconstruction depending on the type of bite.

Differential diagnosis: Part of a syndrome.

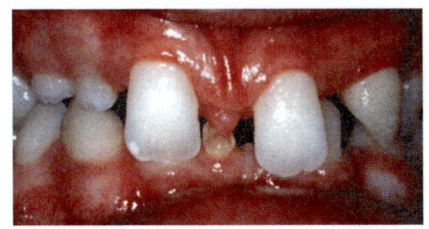

Fig. 18.1.

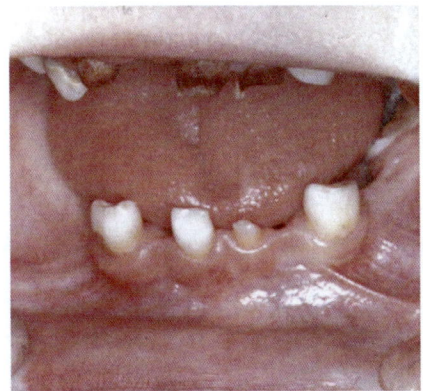

Fig. 18.2.

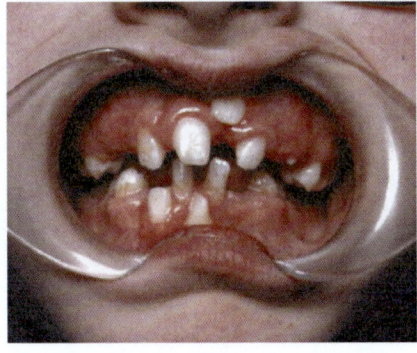

Fig. 18.3.

19. Arthritis – Rheumatoid arthritis

Definition: Chronic inflammatory joint disease, often with extra articular manifestations.

Aetiology: Unknown

Symptoms: Fatigue and weight loss. Joint pain, morning stiffness and impaired movement and deformities.

Orally there is often an open bite in the front and malalignment. Pain and crepitus in the temporomandibular joint.

Clinical features: The disorder often has an insidious course. Starts at the age 30-50. More frequent in women than in men. The prevalence is approximately 1 %. The influence of the temporomandibular joint requires a jaw bone scan which will reveal the destruction of the condyle. 50-60% of sufferers have involvement of the mandibular joints. The juvenile form is often bilateral Fig.19.1.

Diagnosis: Radiologically observable destructions of the condyle should trigger a referral to the doctor for a blood test. A positive test for rheumatoid factor produces a diagnosis.

Treatment: The oral part of the treatment consists of interceptive orthodontics, which seeks to preserve good occlusion. In severe cases, a jaw bone alloplasty should be considered.

Differential diagnosis: Psoriatic polyarthritis, Reactive arthritis, systemic lupus.

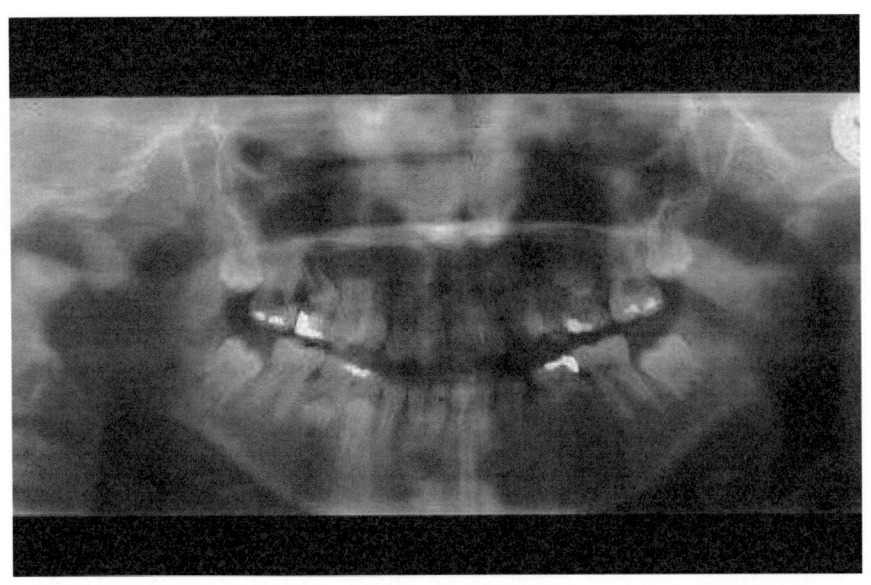

Fig. 19.1.

20. Arthrosis

Definition: Degenerative joint disease that attacks the synovial joints with cartilage destruction, subcondral bone sclerosis and bone formation along the edges of the joints (osteophytes). Also called osteoarthritis or general osteoarthritis.

Aetiology: Unknown.

Symptoms: Pain, both under load and rest. Decreased movement. Displacement and loose joints.

Clinical features: Tenderness, crepitus, restricted movement, instability, muscle atrophy. Can affect one or more joints. Orally there is reduced mouth opening ability, pain and crepitus. Often tenderness on palpation. Jawbone x-ray will show varying degrees of destruction in the condyle and osteophyte formation, Fig.20.1. Restricted joint space.

Diagnosis: Slowly developing joint symptoms. Radiological findings. Fig.20.2 shows a CT scan of the temporomandibular joint with clear distinctions in the condyle.

Treatment: Bite splint, physiotherapy and joint movements, NSAIDs and possibly surgery in the form of joint replacement. Specialist task.

Differential diagnosis: Osteochondrosis.

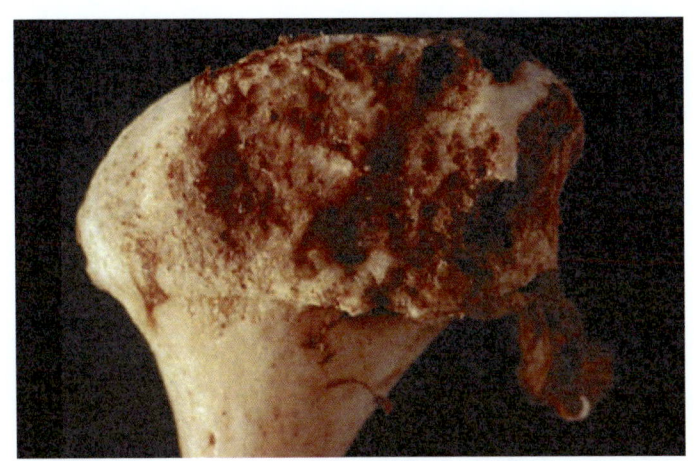

Fig. 20.1.

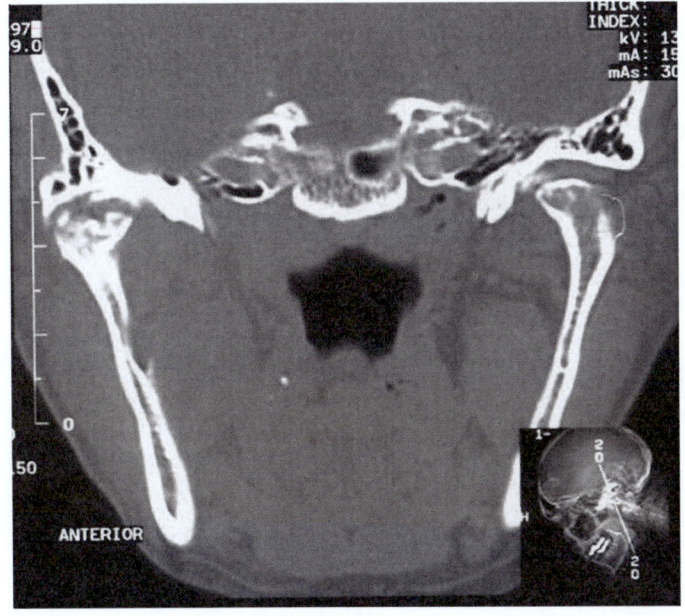

Fig. 20.2.

21. Atrofia processus alveolaris

Definition: A progressive destruction of the alveolar process after tooth extraction.

Aetiology: Tooth loss and lack of stimulation by stress and reduced blood supply.

Symptoms: Hard to get a complete denture for retention. Frequent pressure ulcers.

Clinical features: The amount of tied mucous membrane decreases or disappears completely.

Diagnosis: Performed on the clinical profile and possibly X-ray, Fig.21.1, Fig.21.2.

Treatment: Bone augmentation.

Differential diagnosis: None.

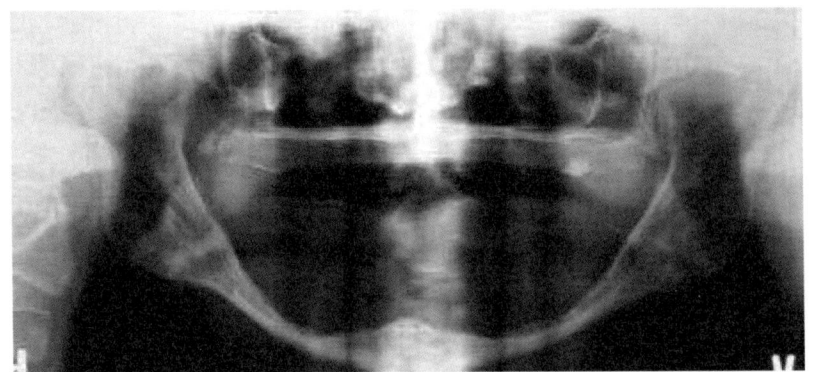

Fig. 21.1.

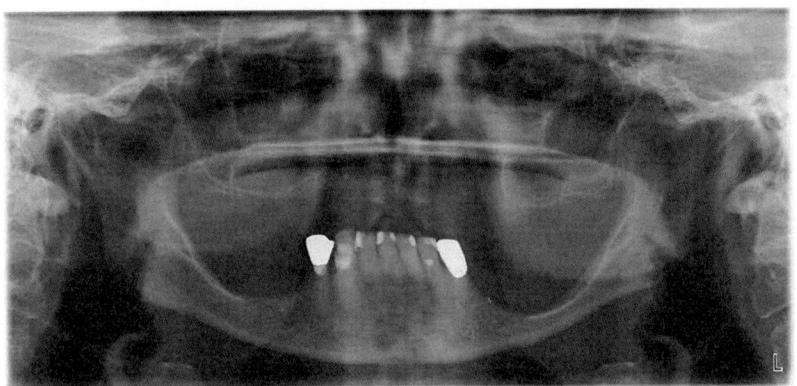

Fig. 21.2.

22. Attrition

Definition: Loss of tooth substance, as a result of mastication. Can be seen both in occlusal and proximal form.

Aetiology: Common natural mastication.

Symptoms: Sore, sensitive teeth.

Clinical features: Wear facets can be recognised by inspection Fig.22.1 and Fig.22.2. Incomplete fractures (cracked teeth) can be seen in the enamel. With bruxism possibly teeth fractures.

Diagnosis: Performed from the medical history and the clinical profile.

Treatment: Treatment is only needed in severe cases. As a prophylactic, a bite splint can be introduced.

Differential diagnosis: Bruxism.

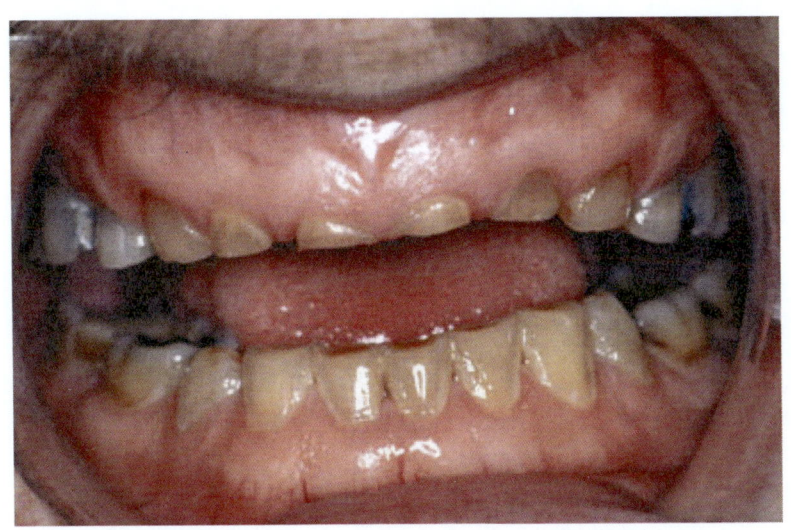

Fig. 22.1.

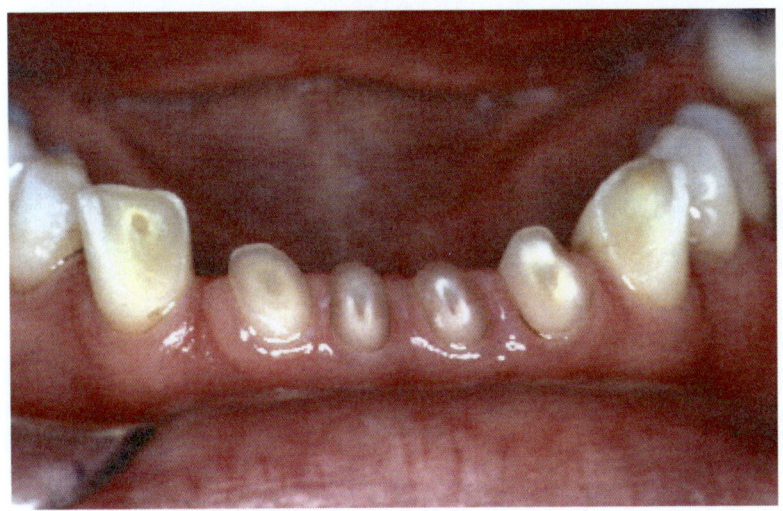

Fig. 22.2.

23. Bad breath, foetor ex ore, halitosis

Definition: Bad breath, foetor ex ore and halitosis are often used as synonyms for the condition that a person has a nasty, smelly and foul smell from the mouth.

Aetiology: More than 90% of cases of halitosis originate from pathological conditions in the oral cavity. This is because of the smelly sulphur compounds hydrogen sulphide and metylmercaptan. In addition, it can be due to circumstances around the tonsils and the area behind the nose and a pathology of the sinuses. If the examination by a dental and ENT doctor is unsuccessful, an internal medical examination is initiated, as diabetes, liver problems, kidney failure, lung disorders and special gastrointestinal disorders may be the cause.

Clinical features: In most cases, bad breath is immediately detected. However, there are some difficult cases where the patient himself can smell a foul odour, but where it cannot be objectively recognized. In these cases, it is necessary to search for a psychogenic cause. Fig.23.1 and Fig.23.2.

Treatment: The dentist must undertake a systematic review of the mouth and teeth. Instruction in optimal oral health is especially important. Purging with 0.1% chlorhexidine and 1% $H2O$ is efficacious.

An increase in saliva production will also help the problem. This can be done by using (sugarless) gum or Xerodent lozenges. Symptomatic treatment can be performed with e.g. Zinc Oral.

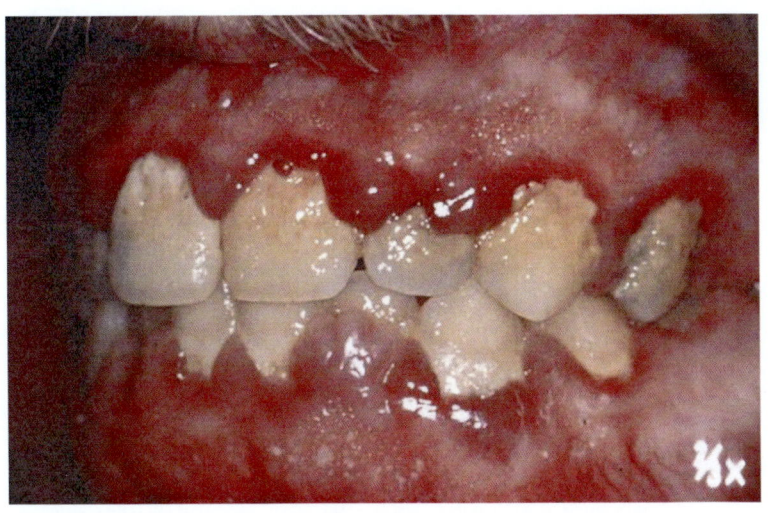

Fig. 23.1.

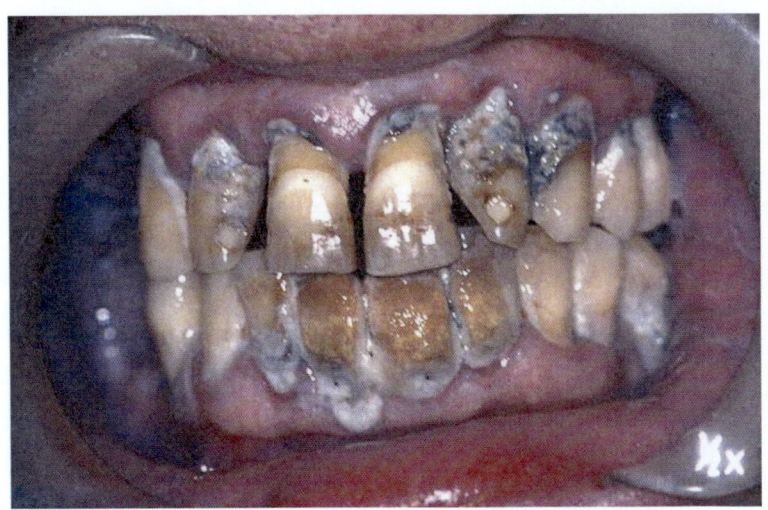

Fig. 23.2.

59

24. Behcet's syndrome

Definition: Episodic, multisystemic and chronic disorder characterised by aphthous stomatitis, genital ulcers, uveitis, cutaneous vasculitis and CNS symptoms.

Aetiology: Unknown.

Symptoms: Oral cavity ulcers are always present, whereas the other symptoms in genitalia, skin, eyes, joints and CNS may vary.

Clinical features: The aphthous stomatitis may be aggressive Fig.24.1 and give reason for further examination by an ophthalmologist, dermatologist, etc.

Diagnosis: Performed on the clinical profile.

Treatment: No effective treatment, but steroid therapy and tetracycline oral rinsing have some effect.

Differential diagnosis: Aphthous stomatitis.

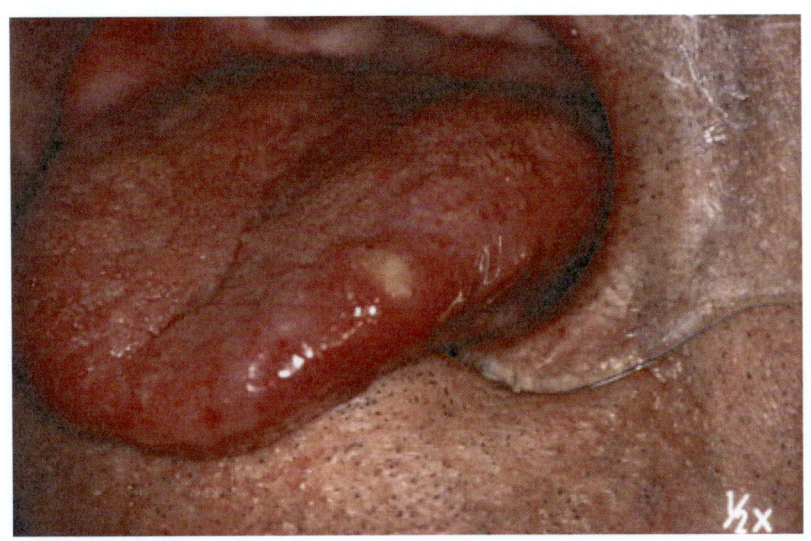

Fig. 24.1.

25. Bells palsy

Definition: Palsy of the 7th cranial nerve, n. facialis.

Aetiology: Often no known aetiology, but the disorder can be triggered by cold and infection.

Symptoms: Paralysis of n.facialis, unilateral loss of facial expression.

Clinical features: Loss of facial expressions Fig.25.1, cannot close eye, blinking or lifting of the eyebrow on the affected side. Angulus oris hangs and saliva leaks out. The eye waters and the face takes on a mask-like appearance. The speech is blurred. Occasionally there is loss of taste.

Diagnosis: Performed on the clinical profile. CT scans can be used to exclude tumours.

Treatment: None known. Most cases resolve spontaneously within hours to weeks, but some are permanent.

Differential diagnosis: Intracranial tumour.

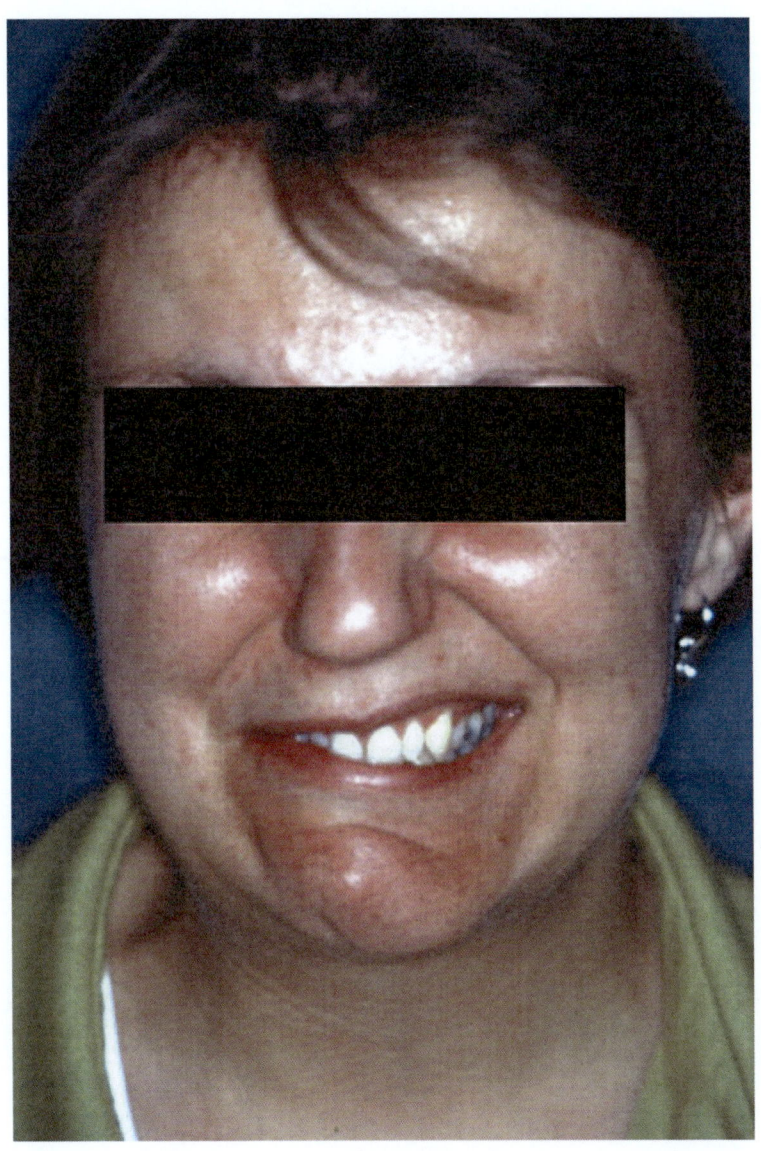

Fig. 25.1.

26. Benign mucous membrane pemfigoid (Pemfigoidea)

Definition: Chronic bullous skin and mucous membrane disorder that mainly affects older people.

Aetiology: Autoimmune.

Symptoms: There are painful ulcers, often fibrin covered, in the oral mucous membrane preceded by skin changes

Clinical features: The mucous membranes has hemorrhagic bullae which rupture rapidly, leaving a reddish eroded area which is then covered by fibrin deposits. The lesions may be extensive. They are mostly in the palate, gingiva, cheek and tongue Fig.26.1. Sometimes changes are seen solely on the gingiva, where they appear as desquamative gingivitis, Fig.26.2.

Diagnosis: The diagnosis is performed by biopsy and immunofluorescence.

Treatment: Diagnosis and treatment is conducted in collaboration with a dermatologist. The general dermatological treatment can sometimes be supplemented with a local steroid salve.

Differential diagnosis: Lichen ruber planus. Pemphigus vulgaris.

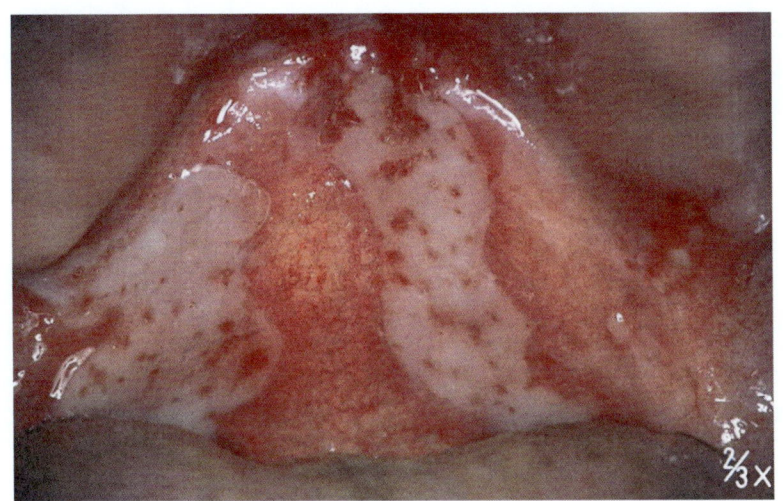

Fig. 26.1.

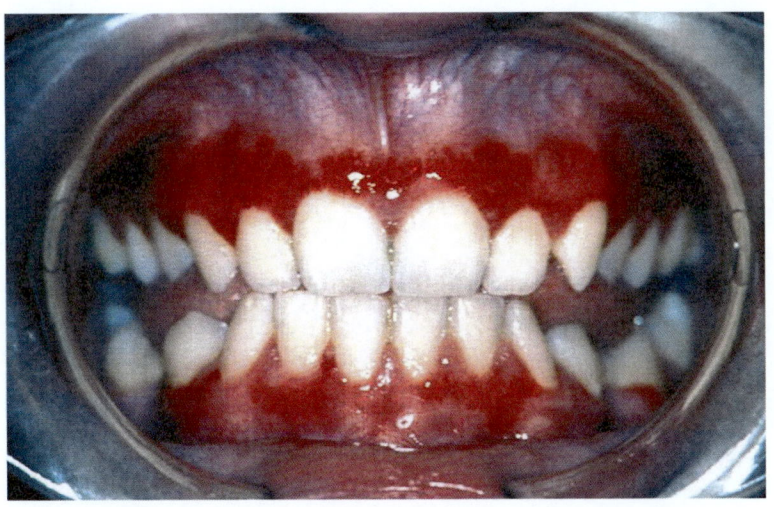

Fig. 26.2.

27. Bisphosphonate-associated osteonecrosis of the jaw (BON)

Definition: Necrosis of jaw bone in patients who are treated with bisphosphonate.

Aetiology: Bisphosphonate inhibits the osteoclasts' resorption of the bone matrix, by which the bone remodelling is inhibited. This results in a reduced elimination of the consequences for micro-damage and thus an increased risk of accumulation of non-vital bone.

BON is only described in the jaw bones (mandible and maxilla). The bone tissue in the upper jaw and the lower jaw is subjected to multiple micro-traumas in chewing. The infection (osteitis) is described as being part of the histopathological image for BON, and furthermore there are findings of actinomycose in approximately 1/3 of patients.

BON develops most frequently after dental surgery (extraction, or surgical removal of teeth), but can also occur spontaneously. In denture carriers there may be a pressure sore from the denture which forms a gateway for infection in the jaw and thereby the development of BON.

BON occurs almost exclusively in patients receiving bisphosphonate administered in high doses iv. as part of treatment for multiple myeloma, breast cancer and prostate cancer.

In osteoporosis patients receiving bisphosphonates in tablet form BON is rarely reported.

Symptoms: In many patients there are no symptoms at first, but eventually there is further swelling and pain and exposed bone.

Clinical features: There are areas of exposed bone with or without inflammation of the surrounding mucous membrane. In rare cases that can be pathological fracture of the mandible. Also submandibular or submental swelling and fistula formation can be seen. In some cases, an additional oral fistula is the first symptom of BON.

Diagnosis: Performed on the clinical history and features.

Treatment: Since oncology/haematology patients are often treated in a major hospital (teaching hospital), where there is a jaw surgical department, they will automatically be referred to it for improvements in the therapy initiated.

During bisphosphonate treatment patients should be checked regularly by their own dentist. Tooth extractions and other bone interventions should be avoided. Painful teeth should be given root canal treatment if possible. If extraction is inevitable, it should be performed in an surgical specialist department. There is no evidence that the suspension of i.v. bisphosphonate treatment before and after tooth extraction reduces the risk of developing BON.

Some recommend treatment in a pressure chamber.

On suspicion of BON the patient should be referred to the specialist department. Apart from long-term treatment with antibiotics, there is no established treatment for BON. In some cases, surgery, possibly with resection therapy, is necessary. Fig.27.1 and Fig.27.2.

Differential diagnosis: Osteoradionecrosis. Osteomyelitis. Radiation sequelae.

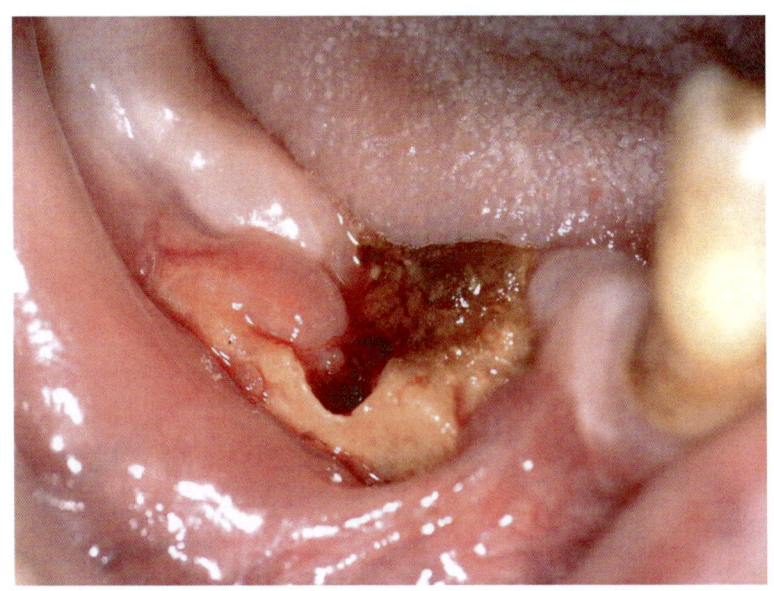

Fig. 27.1.

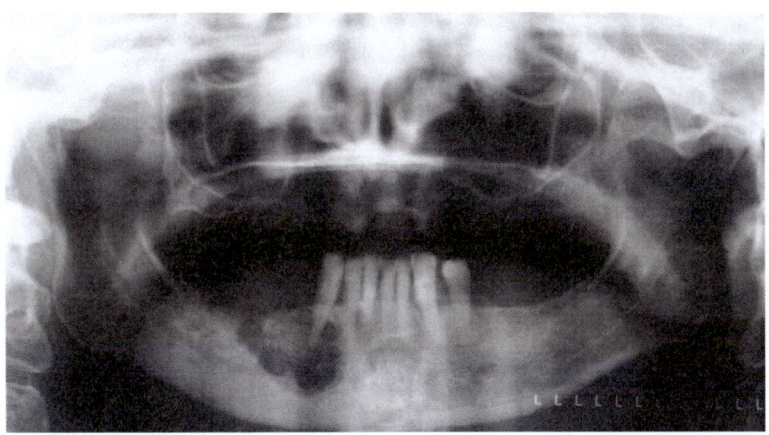

Fig. 27.2.

28. Burkitt's tumour

Definition: Highly malignant B-cell lymphoma.

Aetiology: Occurs in an endemic Epstein-Barr virus form in Africa and in an non-endemic form in the rest of the world. The reason for this is not known.

Symptoms: Dental loosening and extreme swelling.

Clinical features: Most common in children between 3-8 years old. Rapidly progressing and fatal within 6 months. Often swelling of several quadrants. X-rays show large, multilocular destructions. Fig.28.1 show an additional oral swelling. Fig.28.2 shows a swelling in the sulcus, which turned out to be a highly malignant B-cell lymphoma. Fig.28.3 was also histologically verified.

Diagnosis: Performed on the histological profile and special staining.

Treatment: Intensive chemotherapy.

Differential diagnosis: Other jaw cysts.

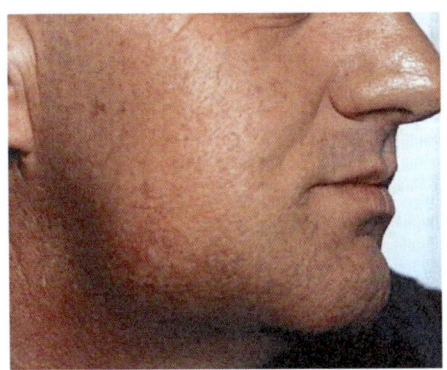

Fig. 28.1.

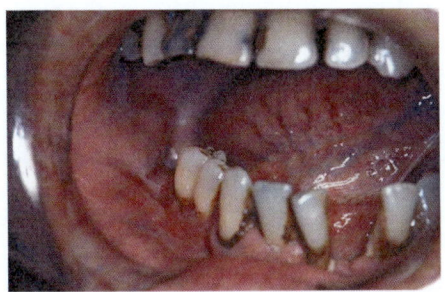

Fig. 28.2.

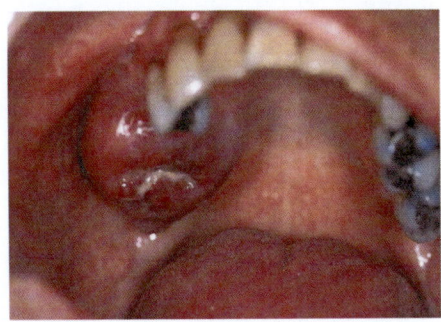

Fig. 28.3.

71

29. Burning Mouth Syndrome

Definition: Atypical pain in the tongue and oral mucous membrane without any objective reason

Aetiology: Unknown.

Symptoms: Stinging and burning in the mouth. Also in the tongue, where it is called glossodynia.

Clinical features: There is a predominance in postmenopausal women. Typically, they have gone through countless studies, but there is no known cause. The mucous membrane is often dry and pale, Fig.29.1, Fig.29.2 and Fig.29.3.

Diagnosis: Performed by excluding the traditional reasons such as Xerostomia, chronic open-mouth breathing, tongue discomfort, mechanical trauma, candidiasis, vitamin B deficiency, in particular B1, B2, B12 and folic acid deficiency, diabetes mellitus and chronic gastritis.

Treatment: Over the counter agents to moisten the mucous membranes possibly with lozenges.

Differential diagnosis: B12 deficiency, and other vitamin deficiency.

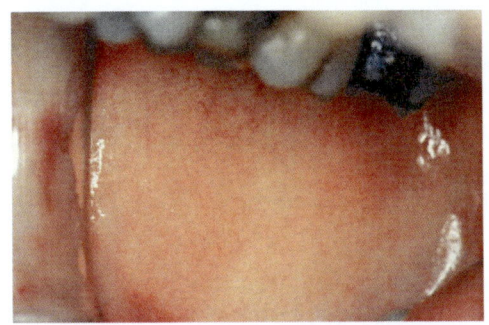

Fig. 29.1.

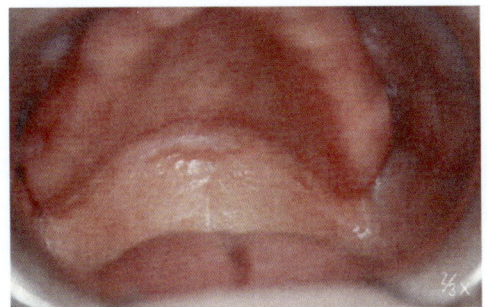

Fig. 29.2.

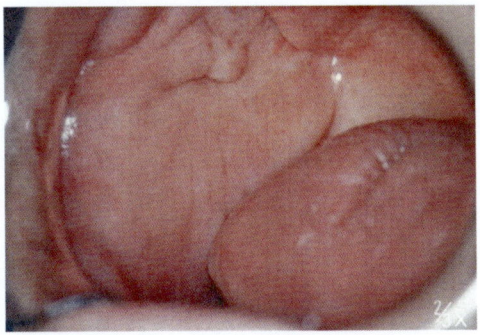

Fig. 29.3.

30. Calculus dentalis

Definition: Calcium deposits on the teeth.

Aetiology: Calcium deposits occur in the organic residue on the tooth surface, called dental plaque. Good oral hygiene can decrease the amount of dental calculus.

Symptoms: There may be roughness on the tooth surface. Dental calculus must be removed professionally. Often, there may be bad breath.

Clinical features: There are large individual differences in the speed with which dental calculus is formed. Also, there is often deposition of soft deposits and plaque, Fig.30.1, Fig.30.2. Dental calculus is also deposited, of course, on dentures which are not cleaned. Fig.30.3.

Diagnosis: Performed on the clinical profile.

Treatment: Professional cleaning. In severe cases, every 3 months.

Differential diagnosis: None.

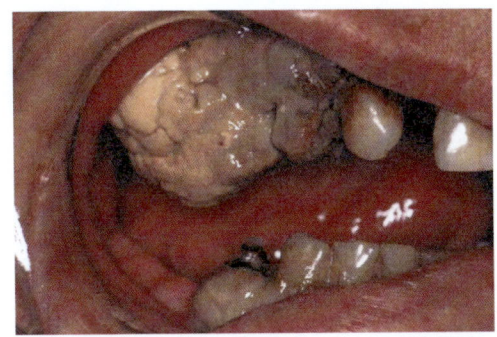

Fig. 30.1.

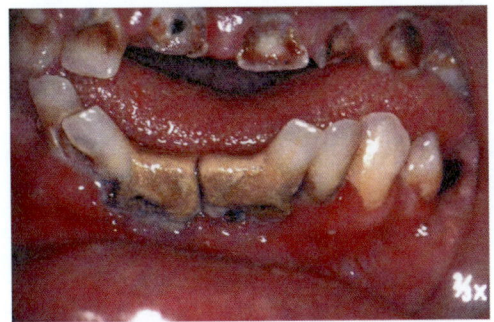

Fig. 30.2.

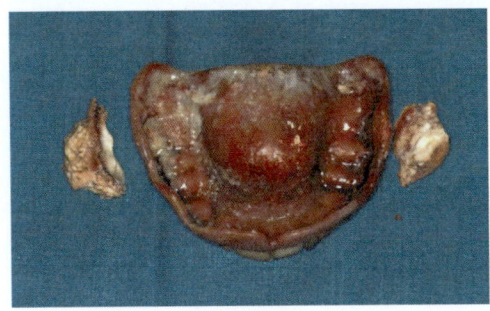

Fig. 30.3.

31. Cancer Linguae

Definition: Histologically confirmed cancer of the tongue.

Aetiology: Unknown, but viruses, alcohol and tobacco are among the causative factors.

Symptoms: Ulceration, which does not heal in 2-3 weeks despite treatment. Also swelling. There is rarely pain.

Clinical features: Insignificant wounds or exophytic nodulations, but often monstrous ulceration or swelling, localised to the tongue side rim and lower surface. The tissue feels hard with rounded sides, typically undermined. The changes in the tongue can be preceded by a leukoplakia. After biopsy, the tissue is disintegrated and difficult to suture Fig.31.1, Fig.31.2 and Fig. 31.3.

Diagnosis: Specialist task. In the event of clinical suspicion refer the patient to university hospital.

Treatment: Will frequently consist of surgery, radiation, or both.

Differential diagnosis: Vulnus morsum, mechanical irritation.

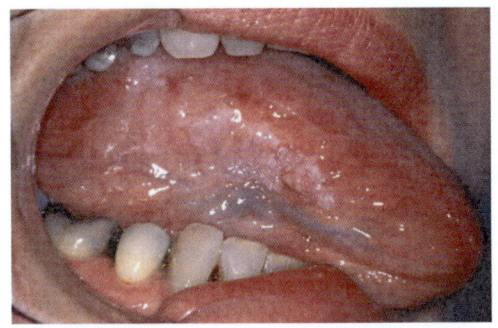

Fig. 31.1.

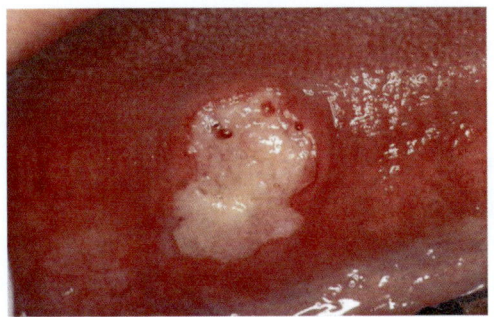

Fig. 31.2.

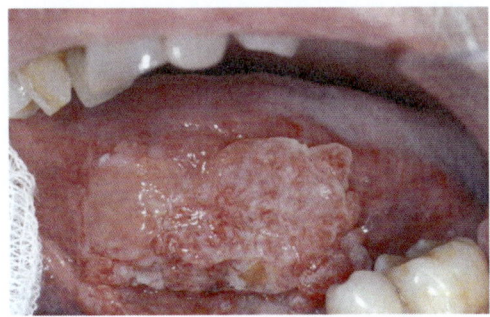

Fig. 31.3.

32. Candidiasis oralis

Definition: An intraoral infection most often with the yeast Candida Albicans.

Aetiology: Fungal infection caused by a local or general reduction in resistance ("the patient's disease").

Symptoms: The acute form produces stinging and burning, and taste disorders, whereas the chronic form rarely causes symptoms.

Clinical features: Oral candidiasis occurs in an acute and a chronic form. The acute form can be pseudomembranous (thrush) or erythematous. The chronic form can also be pseudomembranous and erythematous, but in addition also hyperplastic, Fig.32.1, Fig.32.2 and Fig.32.3. The acute pseudomembranous form is characteristic with creamy leather like, removable white coatings (Thrush).

Diagnosis: By swab and clinical picture.

Treatment: Chronic candidoses are treated for at least 4 -6 weeks, acute for 1-2 weeks. The treatment must often be given both as local treatment for 4 weeks and as general therapy for 2 weeks.

Differential diagnosis: Leukoplakia. Erythroplakia. Hairy leuko-plakia. Lichen planus.

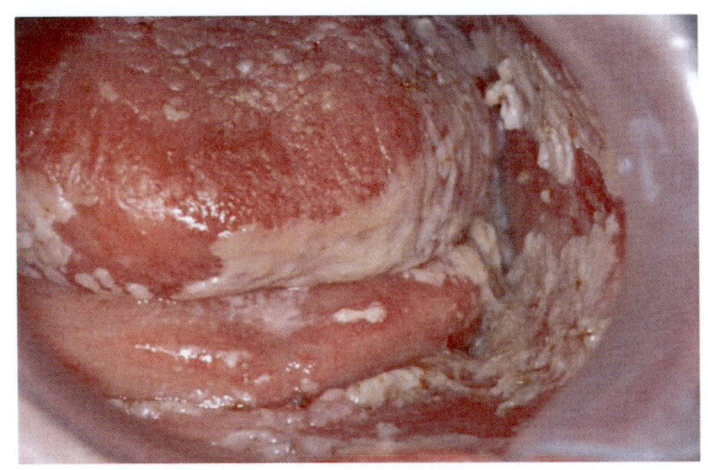

Fig. 32.1.

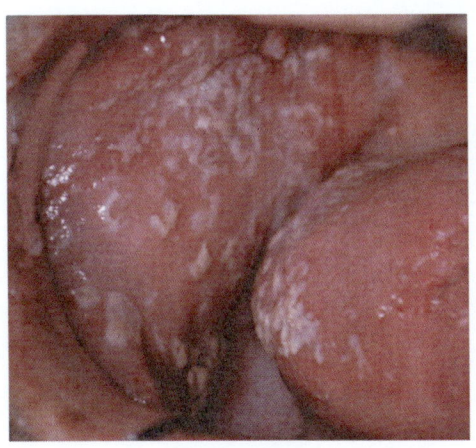

Fig. 32.2.

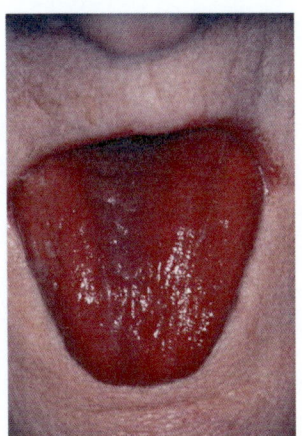

Fig. 32.3.

33. Carcinoma adenocysticum

Definition: Malignant tumor extending from the salivary glands. Histologically defined.

Aetiology: Unknown.

Symptoms: Mild pain, ulcers or swelling with intact surface.

Clinical features: Can occur anywhere, but most often from smaller salivary glands of the palate. Slowly growing, possibly with moderate pain. Either normal or ulcerated surface. If the tumour is located in gl.parotis facial paresis is often seen, Fig.33.1, Fig.33.2 and Fig.33.3.

Diagnosis: Performed on the basis of biopsy.

Treatment: Specialist task. Usually surgery and radiotherapy.

Differential diagnosis: Other malignant salivary gland tumors. Performed on the basis of a biopsy.

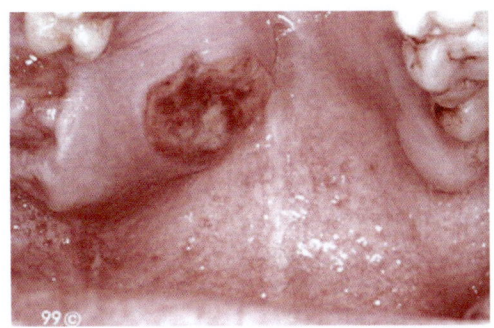

Fig. 33.1.

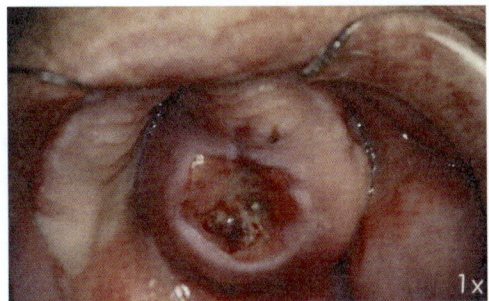

Fig. 33.2.

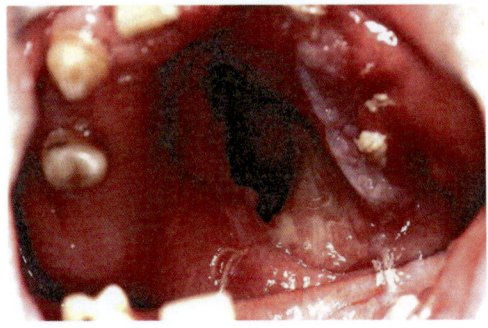

Fig. 33.3.

34. Caries dentium

Definition: Caries, tooth decay, is a bacterial illness that depletes the dental hard tissue (enamel and dentine) and if untreated leads to total destruction of the tooth, often with pain as a result.

Aetiology: 3 factors are required for the development of a hole in a tooth, namely: tooth, bacteria and carbohydrates. The bacteria converts the sugar to in particular acid, in which process the dental hard tissue is degraded. The accumulation of food particles and bacteria on the surface of a tooth is called plaque.

Symptoms: Caries is largely asymptomatic in the initial and medium cases. It is only when the process approaches the pulp that symptoms may occur.

Clinical features: Initially there is a superficial, whitish opacity of the enamel (calcium caries), typically near the tooth neck and on the chewing surfaces. Later there is a collapse of the surface - a hole with a visible defect in the enamel Fig.34.1. A special form of caries is seen after radiotherapy and is called **caries e radiatione** Fig.34.2. and Fig.34.3.

Treatment: Mechanical plaque removal, improvement of home dental care, nutritional counselling and fluoride treatment. Filling therapy.

Differential diagnosis: Abrasions. Enamel hypoplasia. Subgingival tartar.

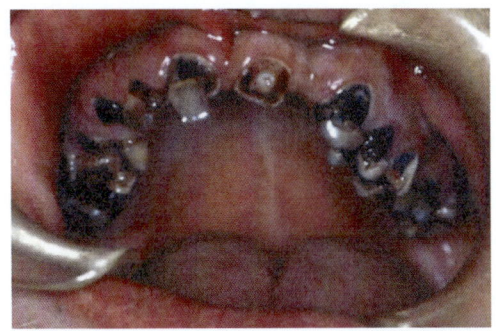

Fig. 34.1.

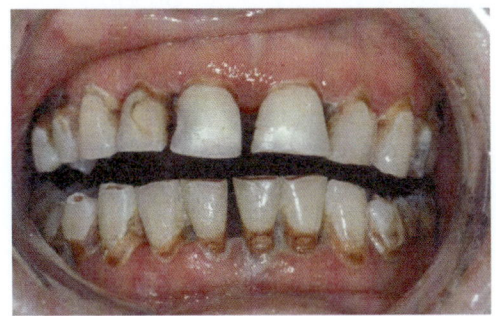

Fig. 34.2.

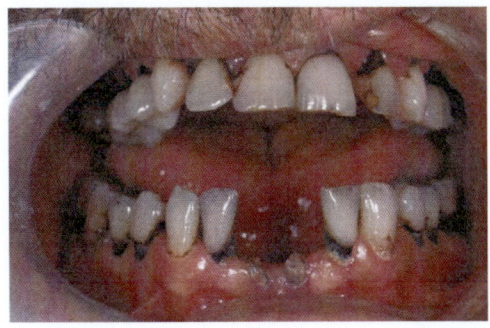

Fig. 34.3.

35. Cementoma

Definition: Accumulation of cement-like tissue around a tooth root.

Aetiology: Unknown.

Symptoms: Most often asymptomatic.

Clinical features: There can be swelling and in radiological terms around the roots of the molars and premolars a well defined radiopaque mass. Often the periphery includes a radiolucent zone Fig.35.1.

Diagnosis: Performed on the basis of the clinical and radiological profile. Possibly after a biopsy.

Treatment: None or surgical removal. Not recurring after removal.

Differential diagnosis: Cementifying fibroma. Periapical cemental dysplasia.

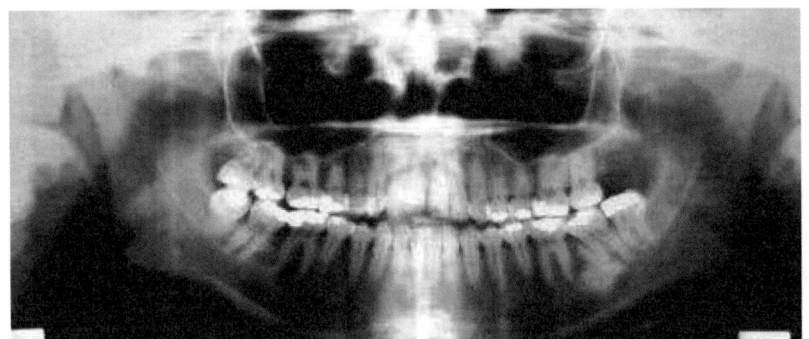

Fig. 35.1.

36. Cheilitis angularis

Definition: Furrows or fissures running in skin folds from the corners of the mouth. Also known under the names rhagades or perleche.

Aetiology: Due to saliva, which flows into the groove. This is seen especially in patients with complete denture or lowered biting height. The moist and warm skin becomes the seat of infection by fungi and bacteria.

Symptoms: There is redness and fissurering of the corners of the mouth and maceration of the skin and pain.

Clinical features: There can be clearly seen unilateral or bilateral furrows from the mouth angle and down, Fig.36.1 and Fig.36.2. Often moist and bright red and ulcerated bottom, Fig.36.3.

Diagnosis: Performed clinically.

Treatment: Treated by antifungals and/or antibiotics. The last after the result of cultivation and susceptibility testing. In denture carriers must the biting height adjusted and the denture base thoroughly cleaned.

Differential diagnosis: Erythroplakia. Iron deficiency anaemia.

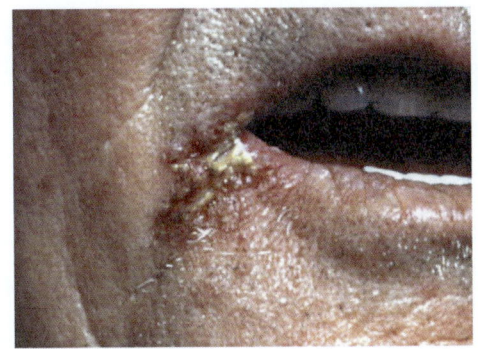

Fig. 36.1.

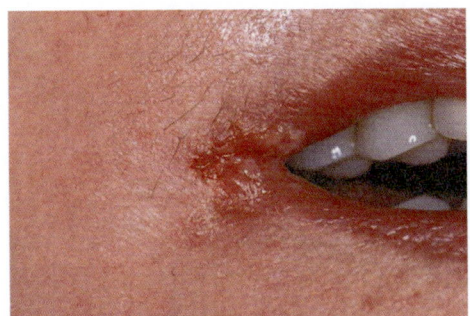

Fig. 36.2.

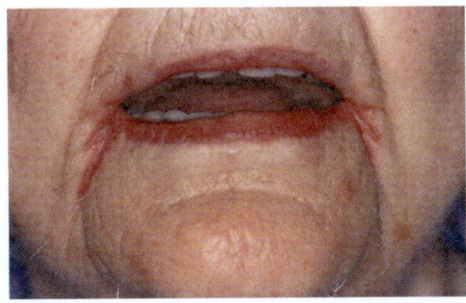

Fig. 36.3.

37. Cheilognathopalatoscisis

Definition: Congenital deficiency, also known as lip-jaw-palate cleft.

Aetiology: The interaction between heredity and environment.

Symptoms: Lactation is difficult voice, eating and swallowing problems. Also cosmetic problems.

Clinical features: The gap is clearly visible and must be operated for 2-4 months age, 2 years age and 12 years age.

Diagnosis: Performed clinically at birth. Fig.37.1, Fig.37.2

Treatment: Takes Performed in a team at the speech Institute. In terms of odontology, the maxillary lateral is often missing in the jaw cleft and treatment is carried out usually at the age of 12. Fig.37.3. These operations take Performed at the National Hospital.

Differential diagnosis: The slots may be more or less extensive.

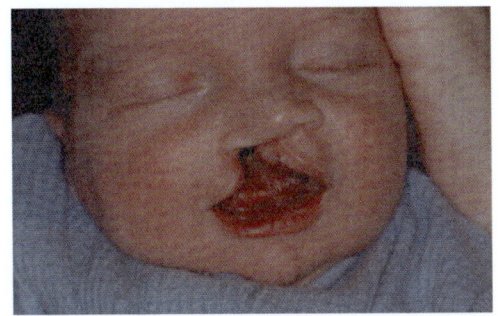

Fig. 37.1.

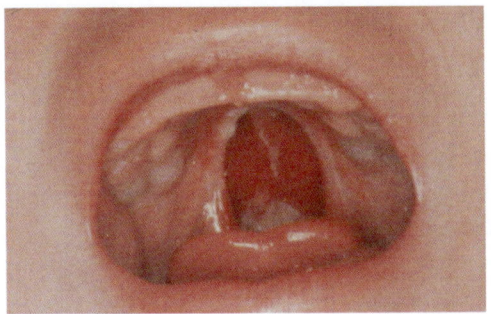

Fig. 37.2.

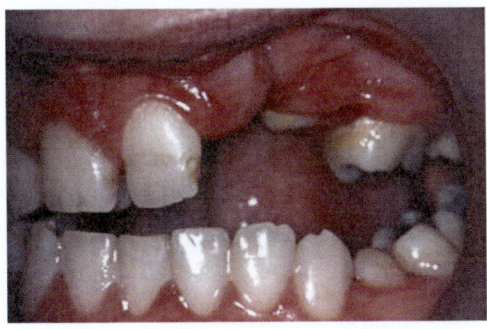

Fig. 37.3.

38. Chondrodystrofia calcificans congenita

Definition: An inherited skeletal disorder that begins before birth. The cartilage is converted into bone, and leads to dwarfism.

Aetiology: Unknown.

Symptoms: Dwarfism.

Clinical features: Damage in the face, facial skin, musculo-skeletal changes. The face is flat, hypoplasia of the malar bone. Forehead prominent with hypertelorism, of mongoloid character, while the nose is flat. Cleft palates can be seen. Fig.38.1

Diagnosis: Performed on the clinical profile.

Treatment: Specialist task.

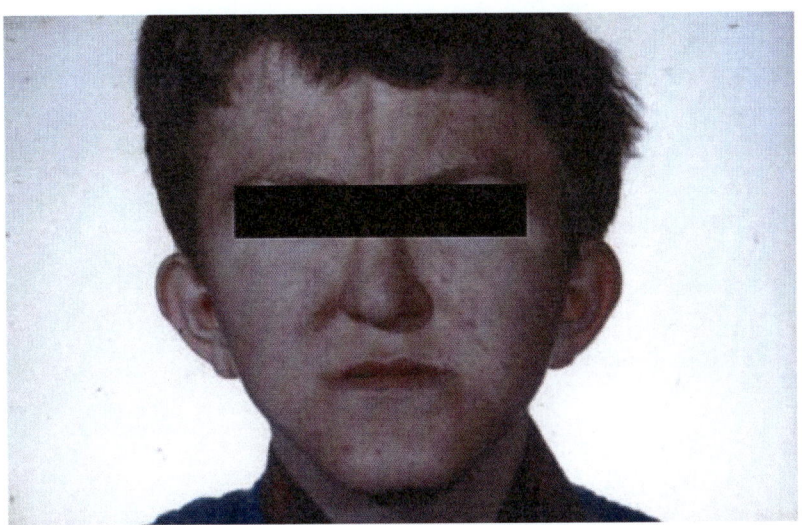

Fig. 38.1.

39. Chondroma

Definition: Benign tumour composed of mature hyaline cartilage.

Aetiology: Unknown

Symptoms: Swelling, pain and possibly dysfunction.

Clinical features: In the oral area tumours are rare, but can be seen around the jaw joint and the front of the maxilla, Fig.39.1. Dysfunction and deviations.

Diagnosis: Performed histologically by biopsy/extirpation.

Treatment: Surgical removal.

Differential diagnosis: Chondrosarcoma.

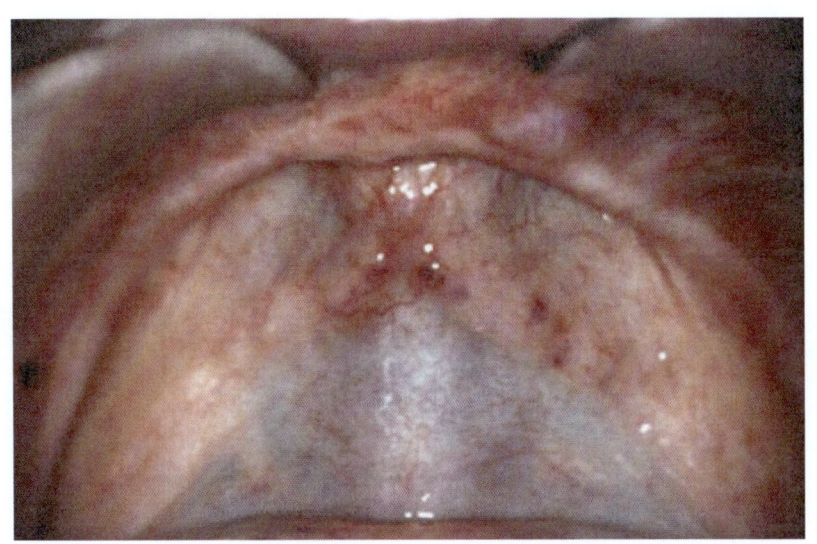

Fig. 39.1.

40. Chondrosarcoma

Definition: Malignant tumour composed of hyaline cartilage.

Aetiology: Unknown.

Symptoms: Swelling without pain. Dental migration and loosening.

Clinical features: The tumour only rarely involves the jaws. It affects all age groups. The average age is 33. Slightly more common in men than in women. Observed equally frequently in the maxilla and mandible and in all locations. In radiological terms there is an ill-defined border zone. There are alternating areas with calcifications and ossification of the cartilage matrix. Fig.40.1.

Diagnosis: Performed on the basis of the clinical and histological examination.

Treatment: Radical surgical excision. Radiation and chemotherapy have little effect. Specialist task.

Differential diagnosis: Chondroma.

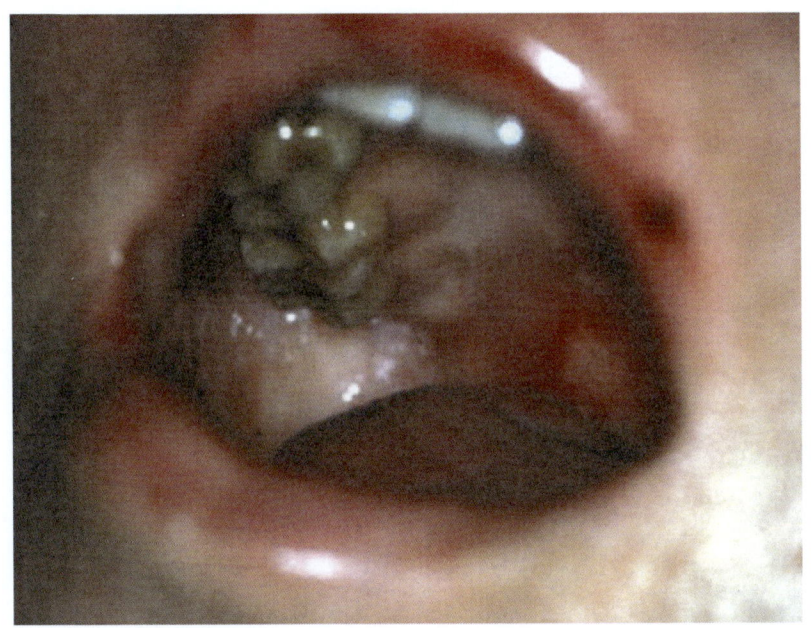

Fig. 40.1.

41. Condyloma acuminatum

Definition: Condyloma acuminatum is a benign, sexually transmitted disease, which is often seen in the ano-genital region, but also can be seen in the mouth.

Aetiology: HPV virus. Usually of type 6, 11, 16 and 18.

Symptoms: No or few discomforts.

Clinical features: The incubation period is 1-3 months. There can be auto inoculation in other areas. In the mouth, there may be one but most often multiple exophytic elements pedunculated or broad-based, especially on the lips, the soft palate and the frenulum. The size can be from 0.5 to 3 cm in diameter. After the introduction of HPV vaccination, it will be interesting to see if the number of cases falls in the future. Fig.41.1, Fig.41.2, Fig.41.3.

Diagnosis: Based on the histological examination and clearance of viruses.

Treatment: Surgical excision or removal by electric cauter. Avoid CO_2 laser because viruses can infect the treatment personnel through the smoke.

Differential diagnosis: Papilloma. Verruca vulgaris.

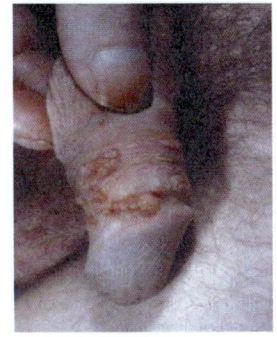

Fig. 41.1.

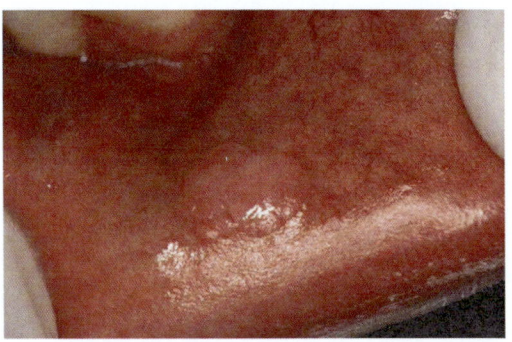

Fig. 41.2.

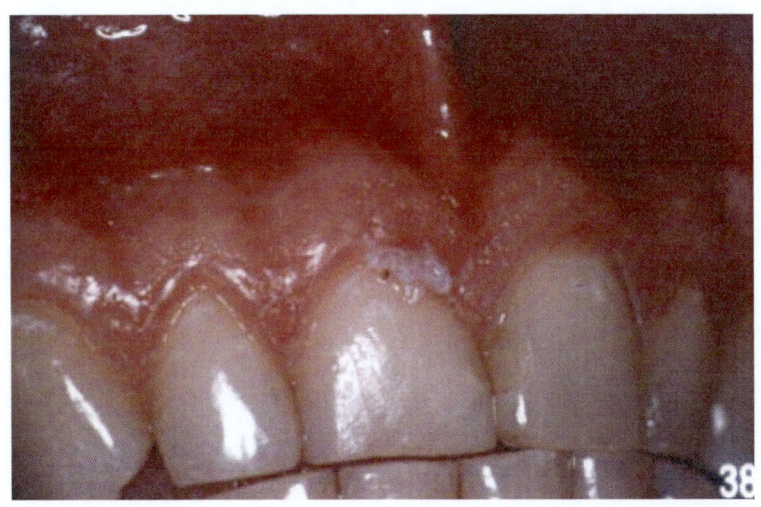

Fig. 41.3.

42. Cysts, intrabony jaw cysts

Definition: An epithelial lined cavity in the jaw containing liquid or semi-liquid material.

The inflammatory-related cysts are by far the most common, making up approximately 90% of all jaw cysts. They are developed from epithelial residues in the periodontal membrane and are caused by an inflammatory process in the periapical area due to a pulp necrosis, **cystis radicularis**. Fig.42.1.

The odontogenic keratocyst is a cyst that occurs in the jaws' tooth-bearing area or posterior to lower jaw wisdom tooth. It is characterised by having a thin fibrous capsule, which is covered by a keratinized, thin multi-layer squamous epithelium. It has a major frequency of recurrence after removal.

It can sometimes be part of **Gorlin's syndrome** which also includes bifide ribs, basal cell carcinoma and a tendency to brain tumour and calcification in the falx cerebri Fig.42.2.

The follicular cyst is a cyst which surrounds the crown and is attached to the neck of a tooth which has not erupted, Fig.42.3.

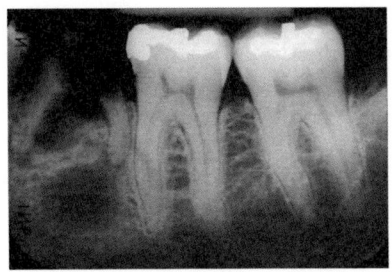

Fig. 42.1.

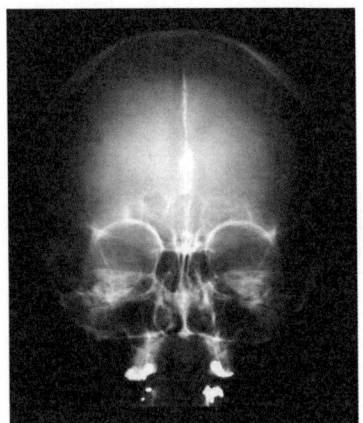

Fig. 42.2.

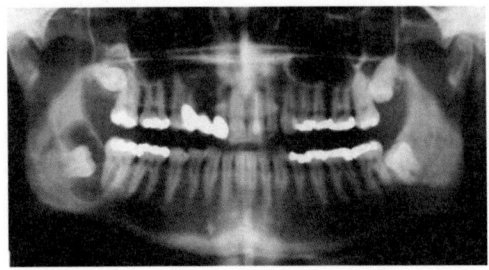

Fig. 42.3.

The Eruption cyst is a cyst covering a tooth which is erupting. Seen only in the primary dentition Fig.42.4.

The lateral periodontal cyst is a cyst which occurs laterally to the or between the roots of vital teeth and which is odontogenetically developed from the residual epithelium, Fig.42.5.

The nasopalatinale cyst is a cyst that has arisen from epithelial residues in canalis nasopalatinalis (canalis incisivus), Fig.42.6.

Symptoms: Jaw cysts are often without symptoms and are typically indicated on an X-ray taken for other reasons. When infection occurs in a cyst, there is pain and swelling.

If the cyst is very large, enlargement of the bone in the relevant area may be seen, and the teeth may also be displaced.

Clinical features: The radicular cyst: In addition to intraoral swelling and displacement of teeth, a radiograph may also show an almost circular, well-defined clearance at the tip of the tooth root.

The odontogenic keratocyst can often reach a considerable size before they are diagnosed by an X-ray where they typically show up as a big multilocular clearance of the mandibular corpus/ angulus region.

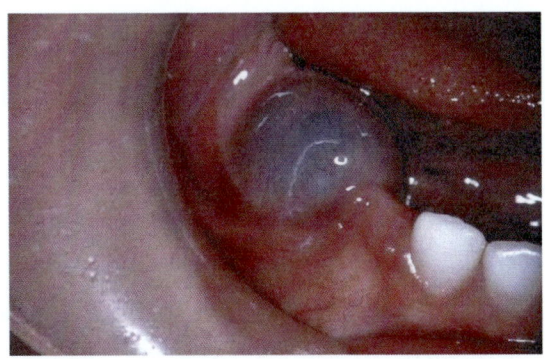

Fig. 42.4.

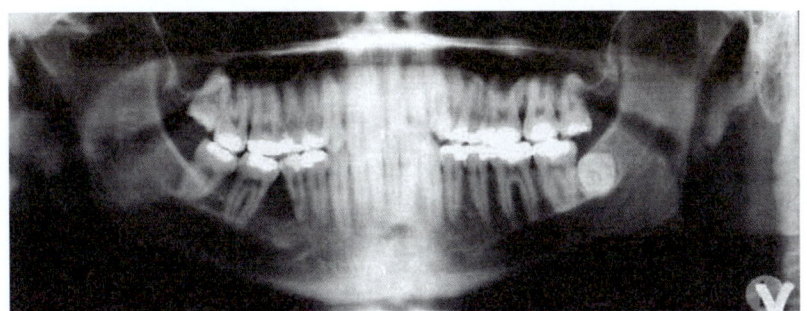

Fig. 42.5.

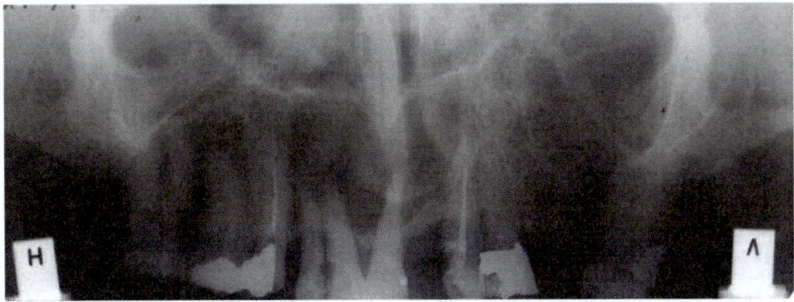

Fig. 42.6.

Diagnosis: Performed clinically, radiologic and by biopsy.

Treatment: There are basically two forms of treatment for jaw cysts: 1) cystectomy, 2) cystotomy.

Cystectomy is a radical treatment with total enucleation of all the cystic tissue and primary suturing. Fig.42.7 and Fig.42.8.

Cystotomy consists of an opening to the cyst with subsequent decompression by means of a small plastic tube and long-term (9-12 months) purging (drainage) of the cyst content. Fig.42.9

Differential diagnosis: intraosseous tumours (especially odonto-genic tumours). Mucoepidermoid carcinoma.

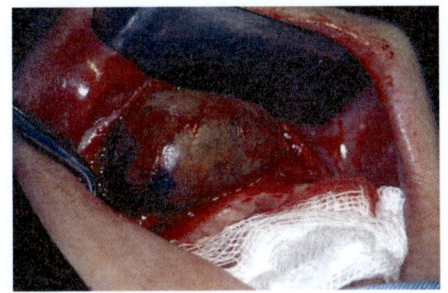

Fig. 42.7.

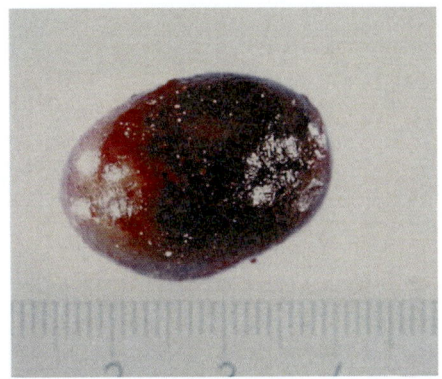

Fig. 42.8.

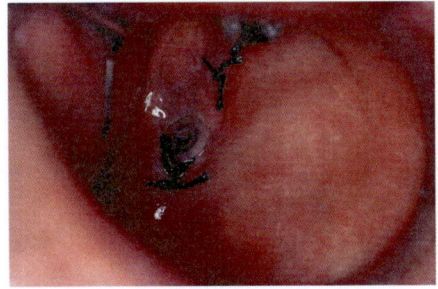

Fig. 42.9.

43. Cystis dermoides

Definition: Developmental cystic malformation.

Aetiology: Unknown. Is thought that, in the germ cells, so-called blastomeres occur that contain cells of all three germ layers – a so-called **teratoma**.

Symptoms: Usually painless.

Clinical features: Most frequently observed in the midline under the tongue. Most frequent in younger individuals. Grows slowly, but can achieve monstrous size, Fig.43.1, Fig.43.2 and Fig.43.3.

Diagnosis: Performed on the basis of the clinical profile, but can be confirmed by a biopsy and histological examination.

Treatment: Surgical removal. Recurrence is rare.

Differential diagnosis: Ranula, Thyreoglossus cyst.

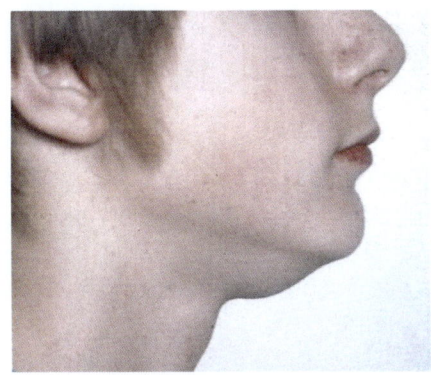

Fig. 43.1.

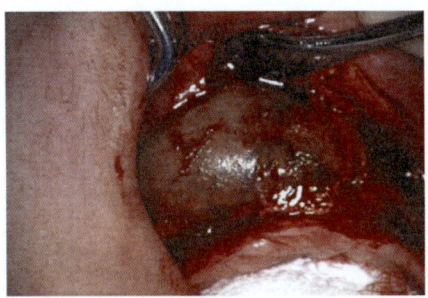

Fig. 43.2.

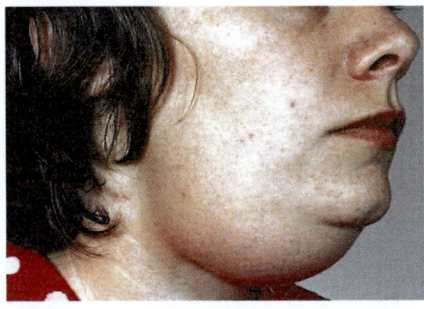

Fig. 43.3.

44. Cystis haemorragica

Definition: Benign, empty or liquid containing intraosseous cavity without epithelial coating.

Aetiology: It is usually considered that the cyst has arisen after a trauma and subsequent bleeding. Also called traumatic bone cyst or simple bone cyst.

Symptoms: Usually none. Swelling and pain may occur.

Clinical features: Seen most frequently between 10-20 years of age. Most frequently in men. Mandible is the most frequently affected. Can be seen bilaterally. Can vary in size from 1-10 cm. The demarcation often goes up between the tooth roots, Fig.44.1 and Fig.44.2. Fig.44.3 shows the empty lagoon intraoperatively.

Diagnosis: Performed clinically and confirmed intraoperatively.

Treatment: Surgical opening. It seems that the opening itself is sufficient treatment. There is usually little or no content of serum-blood exudate. Healing is rapid. At the opening the vascular nerve cord can be seen lying around the cavity. Not recurring.

Differential diagnosis: Aneurysmal bone cyst. Central giant cell granuloma.

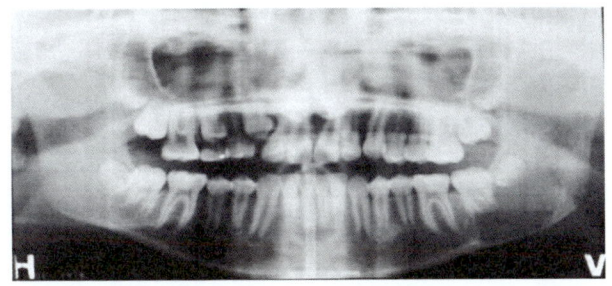

Fig. 44.1.

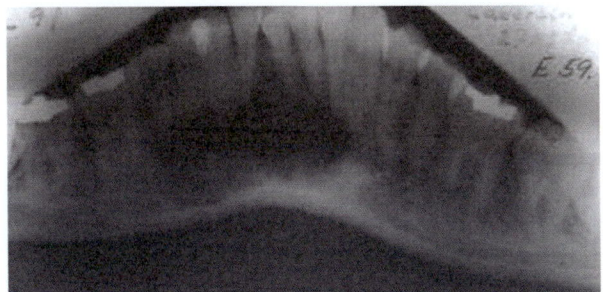

Fig. 44.2.

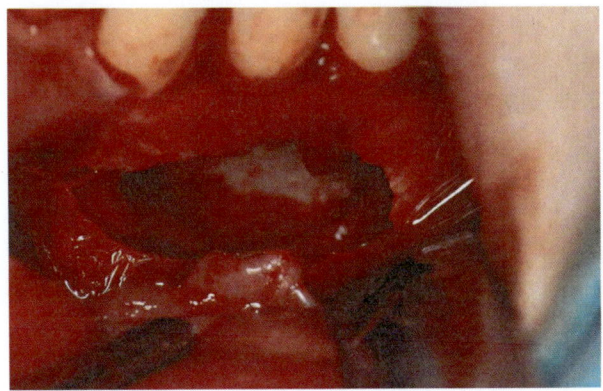

Fig. 44.3.

107

45. Cystis mucosae oris

Definition: Soft tissue cyst, inauthentic cyst.

Aetiology: Can occur by a duct becoming traumatised, typically in the lip, and saliva seeping into the tissue. Also observed on blocking a duct e.g. a saliva stone. In this case there may be epithelial coating and thus a true cyst.

Symptoms: Swelling and functional discomforts. Rarely pain.

Clinical features: Patients will often disclose a bad habit of biting the lip. In the floor of the mouth this can cause irritation before eating. Fig.45.1, Fig.45.2 and Fig.45.3

Diagnosis: Performed clinically.

Treatment: Can be removed surgically or with cryotherapy. With surgical removal relapse is frequent. The patient should be encouraged to stop the habit.

Differential diagnosis: In the mouth bottom **Ranula**.

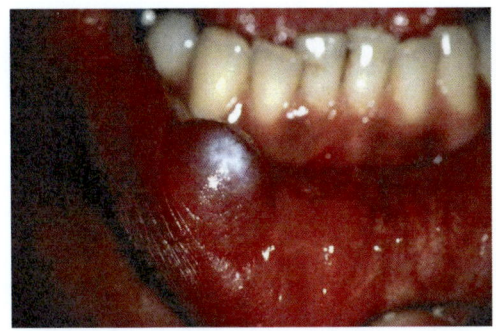

Fig. 45.1.

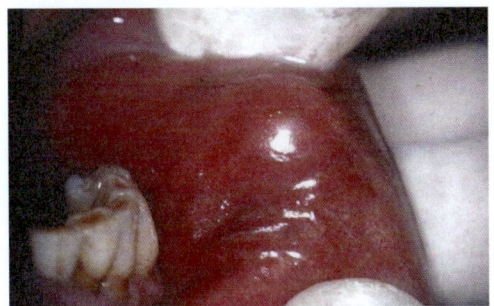

Fig. 45.2.

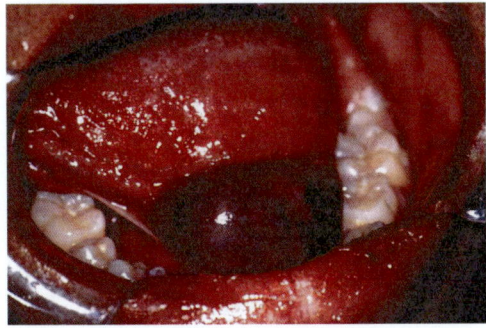

Fig. 45.3.

46. Cystis nasolabialis

Definition: Development cyst, true cyst, soft tissue cyst.

Aetiology: Unknown. The pathogenesis is uncertain.

Symptoms: Swelling lateral to the midline. Lifting the ala nasi. Difficulty breathing through the nose. Rarely pain.

Clinical features: There is a swelling extra orally and in the sulcus alveololabialis. On the X ray it is possible to see an impression in the maxilla front wall. Most frequently in 40-50 years age. Preponderance in women compared to men 3: 1. Fig.46.1, Fig.46.2. Fig.46.3 shows the swelling into the nasal cavity.

Diagnosis: Performed clinically and by the histological examination.

Treatment: Removed by intraoral intervention. Recurrence is rare.

Differential diagnosis: Periodontal abscess. Parulis.

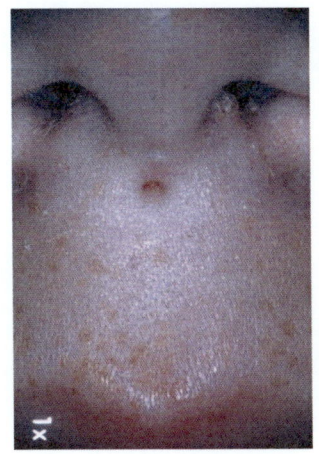

Fig. 46.1.

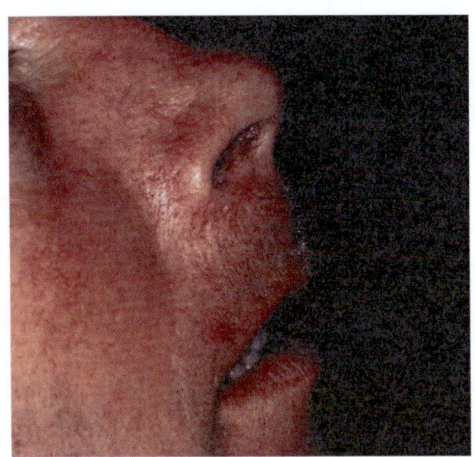

Fig. 46.2.

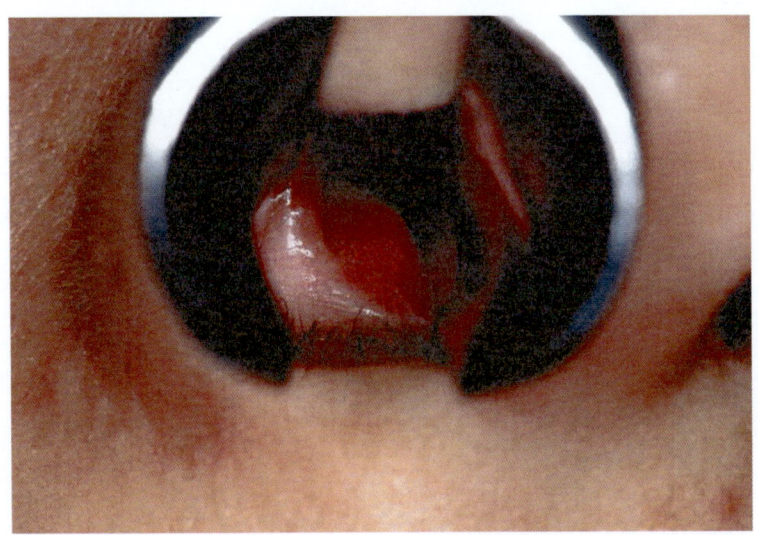

Fig. 46.3.

111

47. Deformatio radicis

Patients receiving radiation during tooth formation can develop deformed and short roots, Fig.47.1

48. Dens in dente (dens invaginatus)

Usually the lateral incisor in the upper jaw. Can cause major therapeutic problems, Fig.48.1.

49. Dental fluorosis

Poisoning of the tooth-forming cells with fluoride, Fig.49.1.

50. Dentes aggregati

Fusion of the teeth during formation. Either the entire tooth or only the enamel Fig.50.1.

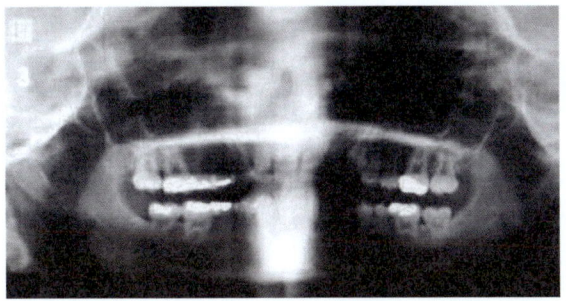 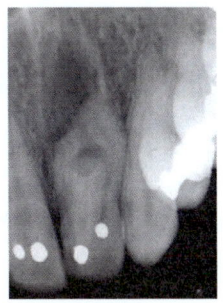

Fig. 47.1.   Fig. 48.1.

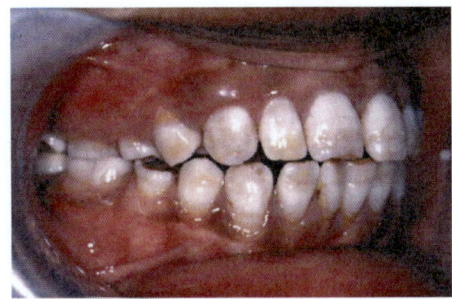

Fig. 49.1.

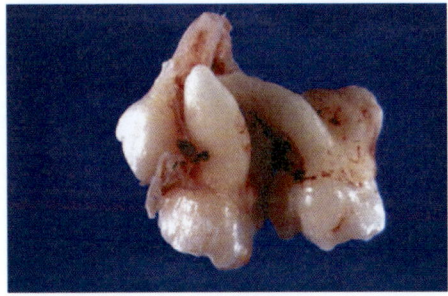

Fig. 50.1.

51. Dentes concreti

Converging of the root complexes, especially maxilla molars, Fig.51.1.

52. Dentes confusi

A total fusion of enamel and dentine, Fig.52.1

53. Dentes decidui persistentes

Primary teeth that persist after normal exfoliation. After removal, the permanent tooth appears, Fig.53.1

54. Dentes geminati

Twin teeth. The fusion can have all degrees, Fig.54.1

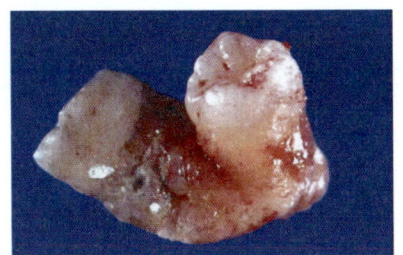

Fig. 51.1.

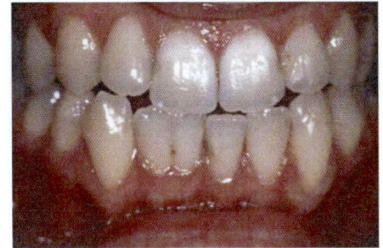

Fig. 52.1.

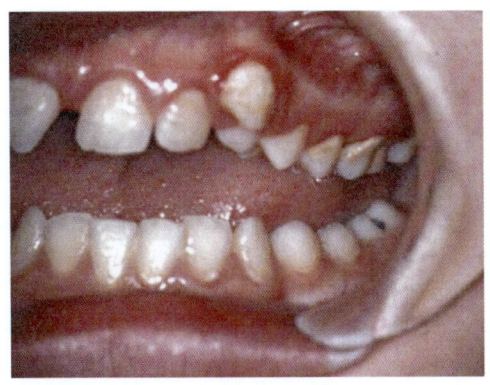

Fig. 53.1.

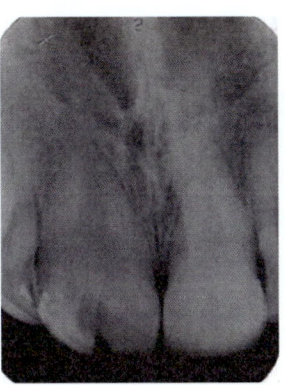

Fig. 54.1.

55. Dentes supernumerarii

Supernumerary teeth are seen in approximately 4% of the population. Most frequently in upper jaw. Mesiodens is the most frequent. Usually creates eruption problems. Surgically removed, Fig.55.1.a.

Dentes connatales, Fig.55.1.b and Fig.55.1.c, and **dentes neonatales**, Fig. 55.1.d., are frequently supernumerary teeth. The teeth are observed at birth (connatales) or within the first 30 days (neonatales).

For the purpose of breast-feeding, it is recommended to remove the mineralized parts. This can be done without anaesthesia because the teeth have no roots. With a "pean", the mineralized envelope can easily be removed. The remaining small pulp polyp necrotizes.

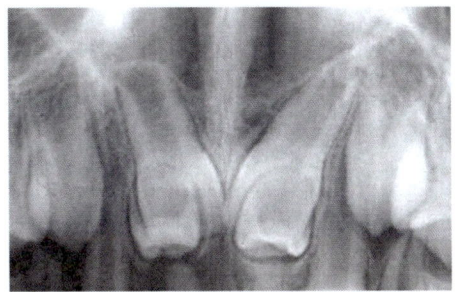

Fig.55.1.a.

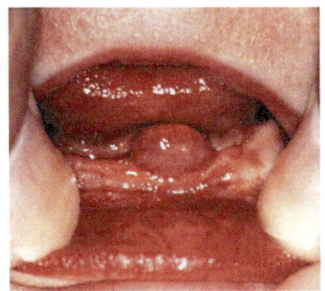

Fig.55.1.b

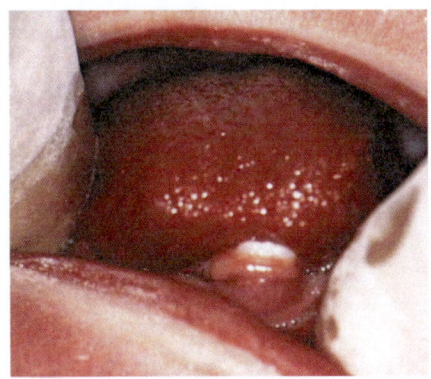

Fig.55.1.c.

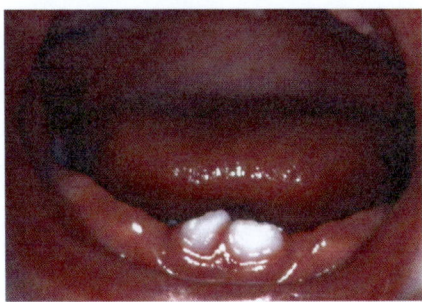

Fig.55.1.d.

56. Dentinogenesis imperfecta

Definition: Hereditary developmental disorder of dentine.

Aetiology: Unknown

Symptoms: Enamel decay and abrasion.

Clinical features: The condition can be seen alone or with osteogenesis imperfecta, which is characterised in particular by blue sclera. It is inherited as autosomal dominant and occurs in 1 out of 8000 individuals. All teeth are affected, both primary and permanent. The teeth have a brown discoloration with translucency. Fig.56.1, Fig.56.2 and Fig.56.3.

Diagnosis: Performed on the clinical profile and medical history.

Treatment: Early crown treatment of the first molar is important for maintaining the biting height. Energetic prophylaxis. Cosmetic prosthetics.

Differential diagnosis: Tetracyclin discoloration, Amelogenesis imperfecta.

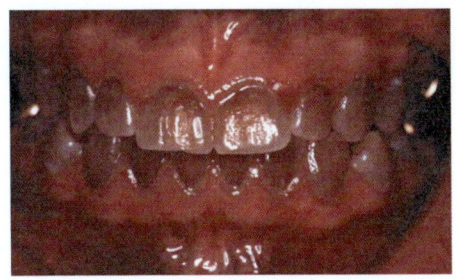

Fig. 56.1.

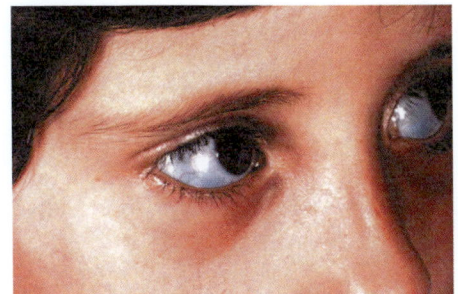

Fig. 56.2.

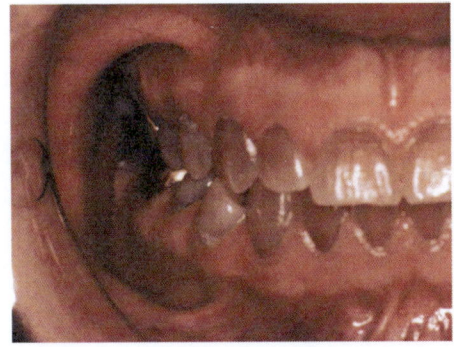

Fig. 56.3.

57. Dentitio difficilis

Difficult teething. Often, pain and infection. Surgical intervention is often required, Fig.57.1.

58. Dentitio tarda

Delayed tooth formation. Rarely in the primary dentition, frequently in the permanent dentition. A general delayed onset may be due to nutritional deficiencies, endocrinopathies or chromosomal abnormalities. For each tooth it is necessary to consider local obstacles, Fig.58.1.

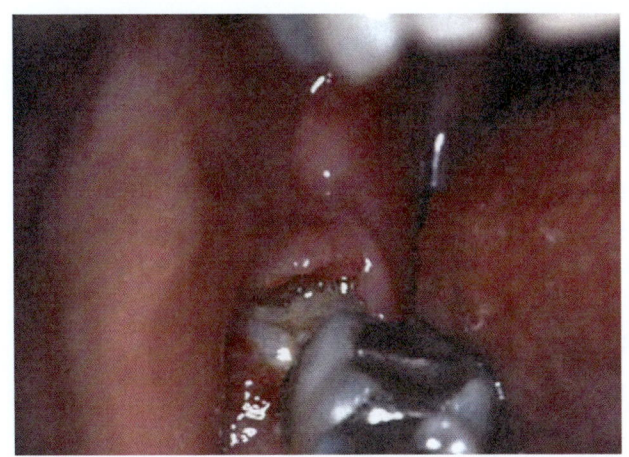

Fig. 57.1.

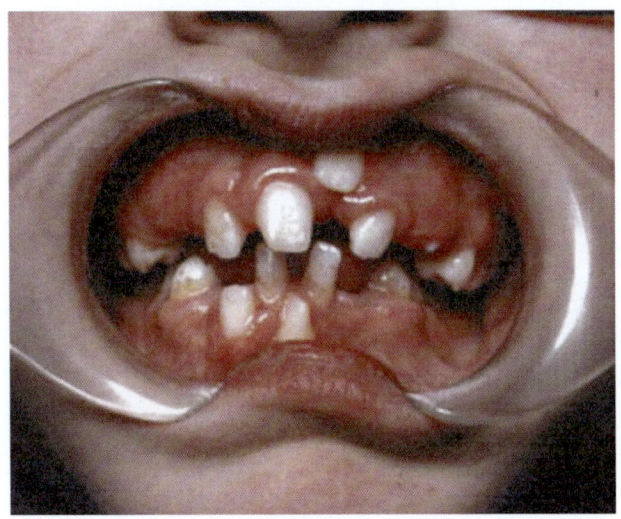

Fig. 58.1.

59. Denture-related mucosal disease

Ulcus Decubitale

Definition: Pathological changes in the oral mucous membrane caused by poorly fitting dentures.

Aetiology: Poorly fitted dentures.

Symptoms: Pain on touch and use of the denture. Wounds in the mucous membrane.

Clinical features: Pressure ulcers are most commonly seen in the sulcus facially or orally for the alveolar proces. The ulcerations are fibrin coated, often with accented edges, giving them a suspicious appearance, Fig.59.1.

Diagnosis: Performed from the medical history and the clinical profile.

Treatment: Decompres the denture. Possibly rebasing, duplication or new production. If the ulcer persists despite treatment, then take a biopsy.

Differential diagnosis: C. oris.

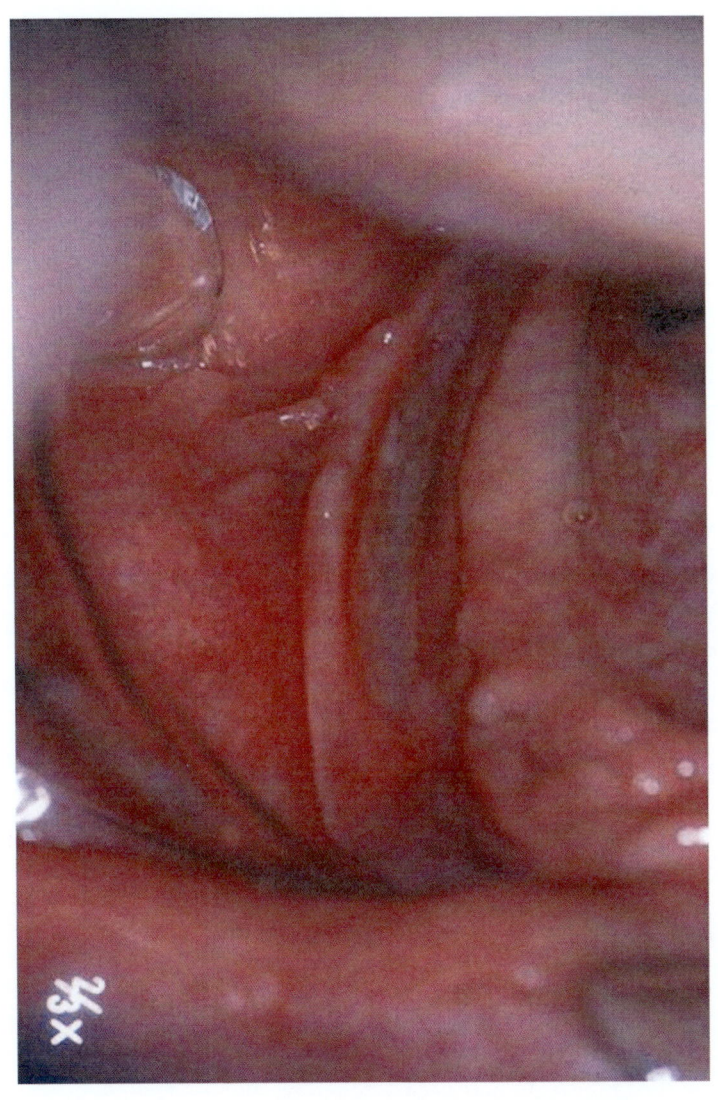

Fig. 59.1.

Hyperplasia Irritationis

Definition: Pathological changes in the oral mucous membrane caused by poorly fitting dentures.

Aetiology: The fibrotic tissue is a repair response to small wounds and maladaptive dentures.

Symptoms: The patient complains of unstable dentures and "sausage -shaped" tissue masses in the mouth. Bad breath and recurrent ulcerations.

Clinical features: The mucous membrane hyperplasias consist of solid, fibrous connective tissue, localised to the alveolar ridge, or facially or orally present. In terms of size, they can vary from less than one cm to monstrous tumour-like masses, Fig.59.2 and Fig.59.3.

Diagnosis: Performed from the medical history, clinical findings and possibly a biopsy.

Treatment: Surgery, prosthetic treatment and antifungal treatment.

Differential diagnosis: None.

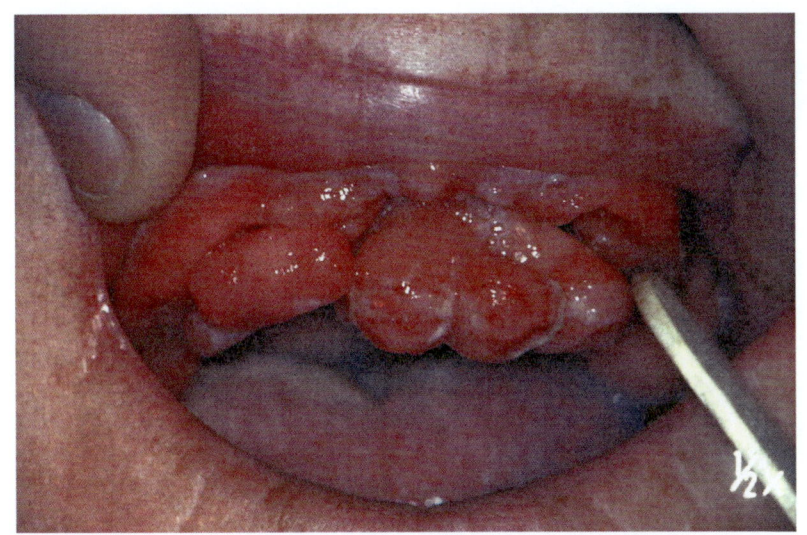

Fig. 59.2.

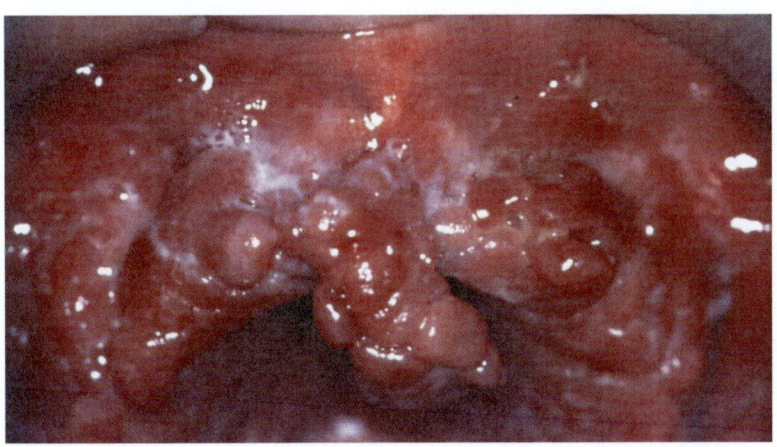

Fig. 59.3.

Stomatitis prothetica

Definition: Fiery red mucosa under the prothesis.

Symptoms: None or a few subjective symptoms.

Clinical features: There is intense redness under the denture base. In the palate, there may be less localised areas or the entire palate may be involved. Sometimes you will find a nodular hyperplastic thickening of the palatine mucous membrane. The condition is almost always associated with chronic candidiasis, Fig.59.4.

Diagnosis: Performed clinically, smears for fungi.

Treatment: The hyperplasias must be surgically removed. Any prothesestomatites require antifungal treatment. It is important that the denture be treated simultaneously. If there are nodular hyperplasias in the palate, they must also be removed. Finally, there must be an alignment of the denture (grinding, rebasing, duplication), or production of a new one.

Differential diagnosis: Carcinoma. Allergy to denture material. Other tumour.

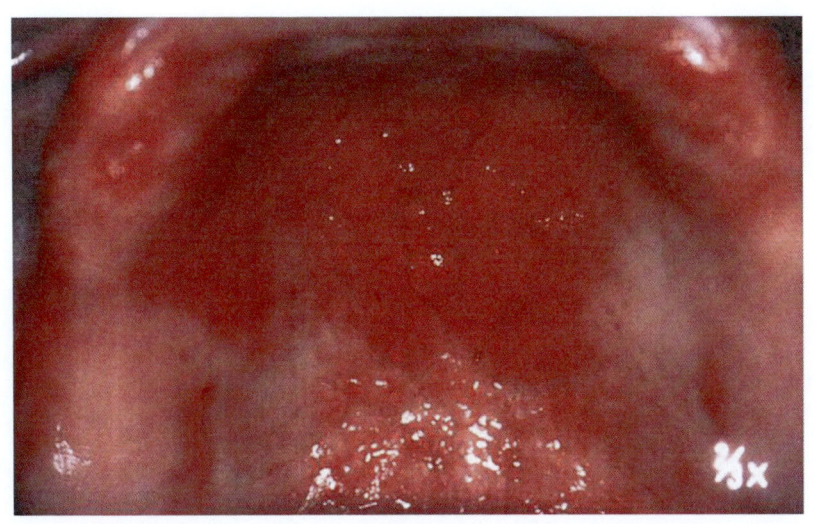

Flg. 59.4.

60. Dermatitis herpetiformis

In connection with a Zoster infection there is frequently affection of the skin. Fig.60.1.

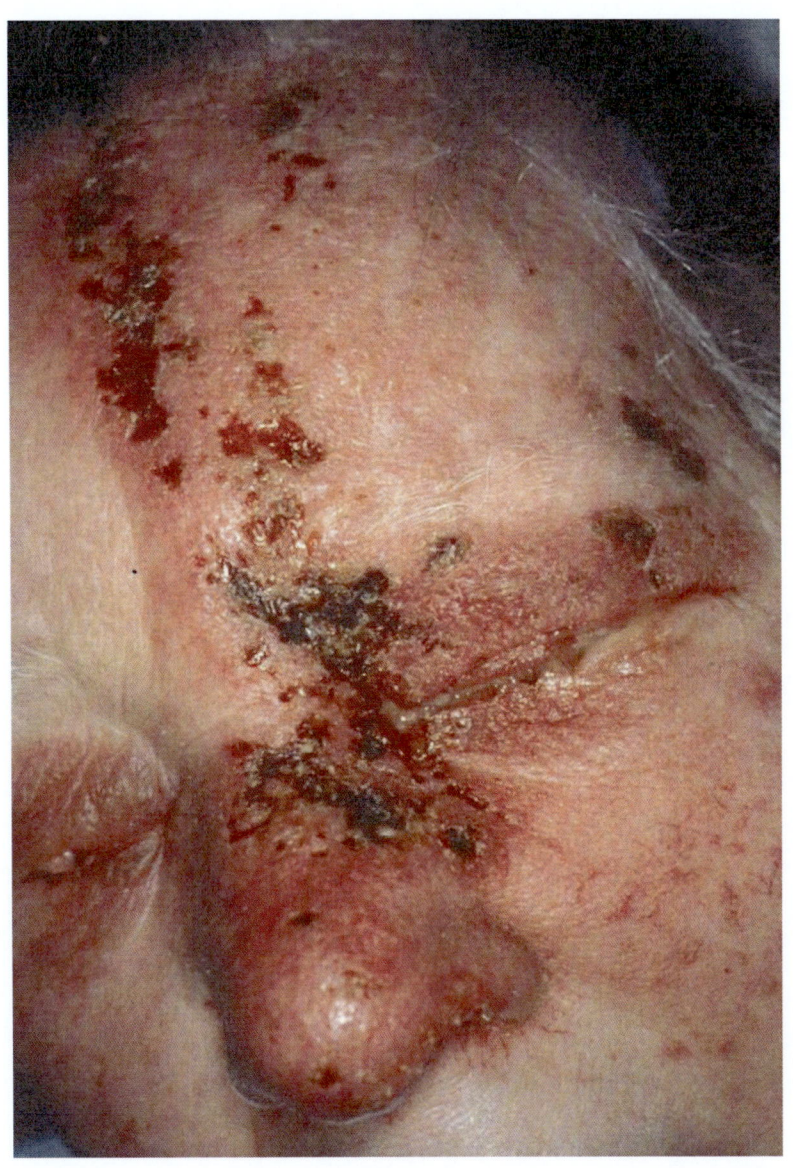

Fig. 60.1.

61. Discoloratio dentis

Definition: Colour change of the tooth's natural colour, either **exogenous** or **endogenous**.

Aetiology: The reason can be trauma, medicine during tooth formation, tobacco, red wine, etc.

Symptoms: None.

Clinical features: In conjunction with a trauma, the pulp may necrose and the necrotic waste products will produce a greyish colour. A thorough medical history will clarify any medication. Fig.61.1, Fig.61.2, Fig.61.3.

Diagnosis: Performed clinically and from the medical history.

Treatment: Root canal treatment, cosmetic prosthetics.

Differential diagnosis: None.

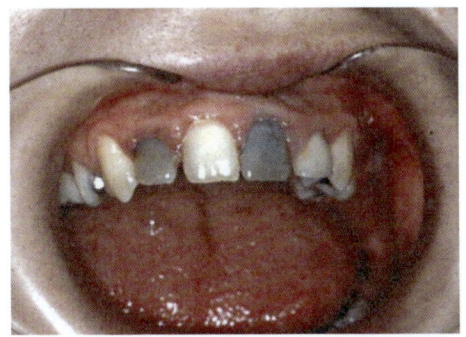

Fig. 61.1.

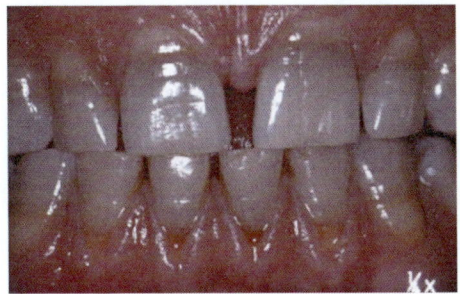

Fig. 61.2.

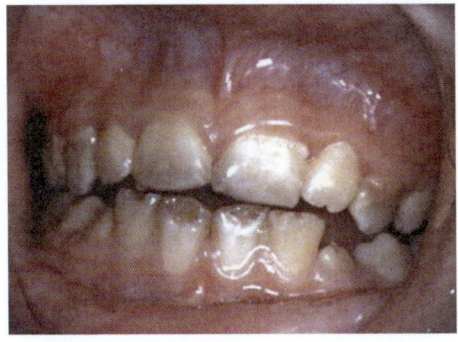

Fig. 61.3.

62. Discoloratio mucosae oris

Definition: Change of the colour from the normal mucous membrane.

Aetiology: The cause may be endogenous or exogenous. For example, antimalarials, tranquillisers, Cisplatin and oral contraceptives. Also, tobacco, amalgam and pathologies, e.g. freckle or melanoma.

Symptoms: Asymptomatic.

Clinical features: Pigmentations without a historical cause must be observed and possibly referred to a specialist unit for assessment and biopsy. Fig.62.1, Fig.62.2. Also Fig.62.3 which was a malignant melanoma. The intraoral malignant melanoma is extremely rare and accounts for only 1% of malignant melanomas, but the prognosis is very poor.

Diagnosis: Most often the medical history produces a diagnosis, alternatively histological examination.

Treatment: The condition requires no treatment in most cases. Suspicion of melanoma requires referral.

Differential diagnosis: Ethnic pigmentation.

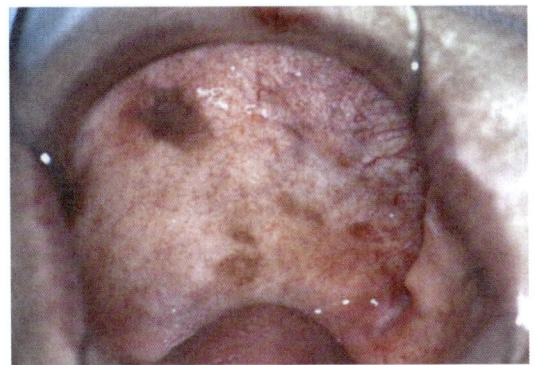
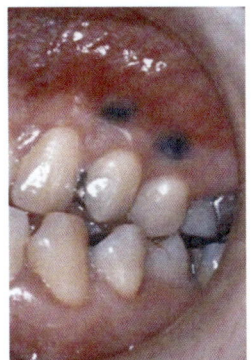

Fig. 62.1.   Fig. 62.2.

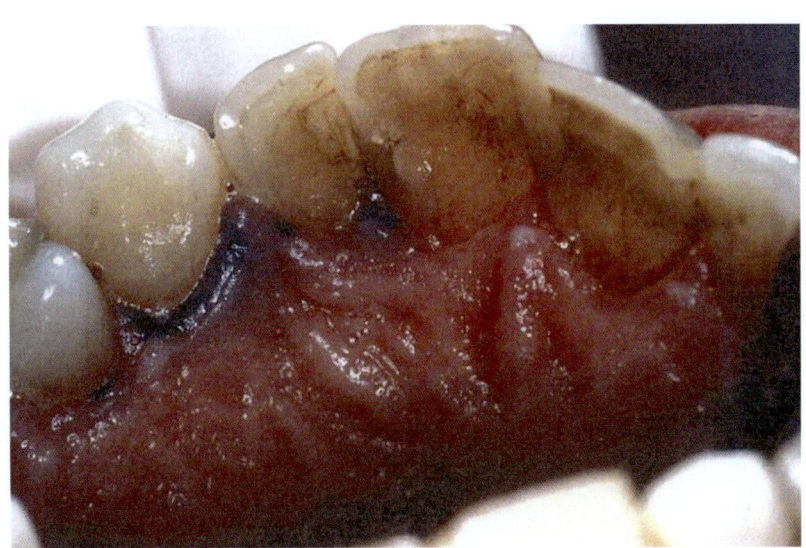

Fig. 62.3.

63. Dysostosis cleidocranialis

Definition: Malformations in claviculae and skull.

Aetiology: Genetic defect

Symptoms: Low growth.

Clinical features: Patients show lack of growth and lack of claviculae, possibly with hypoplasia. Mentally normal. The disorder is inherited. The skull is wide. Frontal bossing. Maxilla is poorly developed. Dentitio tarda and lack of dropping of the primary teeth. Multiple retentions and supernumerary teeth. The condition is requiring treatment. Fig.63.1, Fig.63.2. and Fig.63.3.

Diagnosis: Chromosome study and history.

Treatment: Requires prolonged treatment until growth is completed.

Differential diagnosis: Other osteodysplasias.

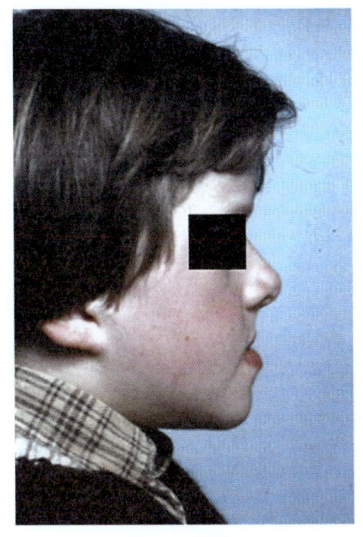 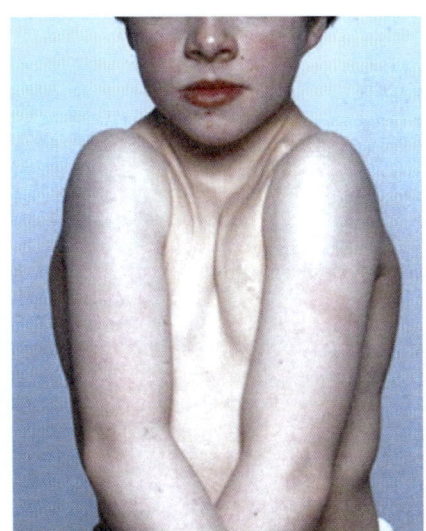

Fig. 63.1.   Fig. 63.2.

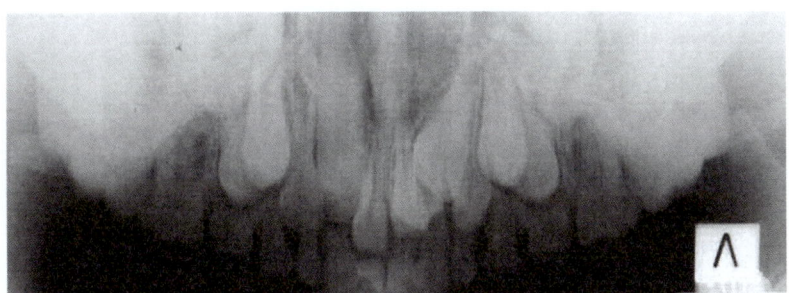

Fig. 63.3.

135

64. Dysplasia ectodermalis

Definition: Dysplasia in ectodermally derived tissue.

Aetiology: Genetic defect.

Symptoms: None.

Clinical features: Prominent tubera frontalis and saddle nose. Hair, eyelashes and eyebrows are sparse and white. Inability to sweat, nails are spoon-shaped. Intraorally there can be hypodontia, anodontia and delayed tooth eruption. The teeth have a simple conical shape. Fig.64.1 and Fig.64.2 and Fig.64.3.

Diagnosis: Performed in consultation with the patient's physician and possibly a genetic laboratory.

Treatment: Very complex and lifelong treatment of dental problems.

Differential diagnosis: Chondroectodermal dysplasia.

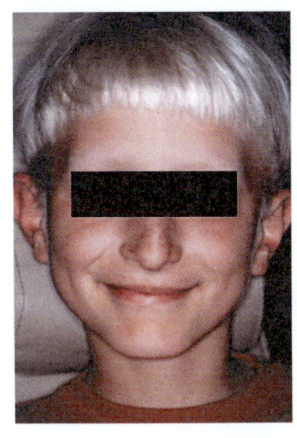

Fig. 64.1.

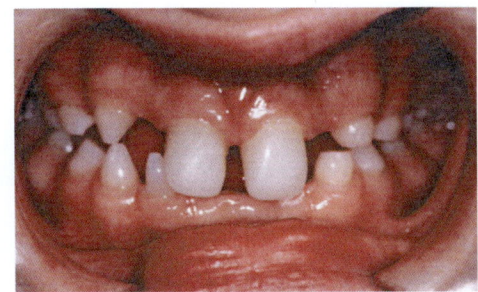

Fig. 64.2.

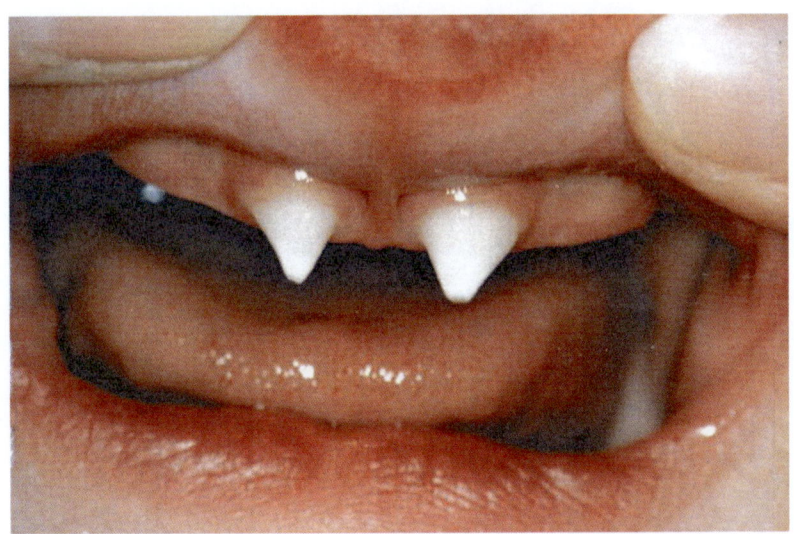

Fig. 64.3.

65. Dysplasia fibrosa

Definition: Benign condition characterised by fibrous connective tissue containing trabeculae of immature bone.

Aetiology: Unknown, genetic mutation.

Symptoms: Swelling, rarely pain.

Clinical features: Slow-growing swelling without pain. Periods of accelerated swelling and asymmetry. The disease starts early and fades away in many cases after puberty. Can be found in 2 forms Monoostotic and Polyostotic (Albright's syndrome). The jaws are always involved. Maxilla slightly higher than the mandible, Fig.65.1. Somewhat more frequently in women than in men. Radiologically the disorder looks like frosted glass. Cherubism is referred to as familial fibrous dysplasia, Fig.65.2, Fig.65.3.

Diagnosis: Clinical profile and biopsy with histology.

Treatment: As appropriate. Possibly cosmetic corrections referred to a specialised department.

Differential diagnosis: Other fibro-osseous disorders.

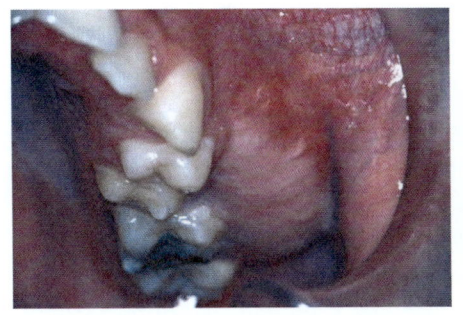 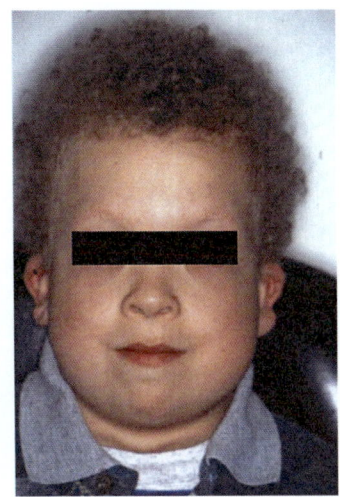

Fig. 65.1.   Fig. 65.2.

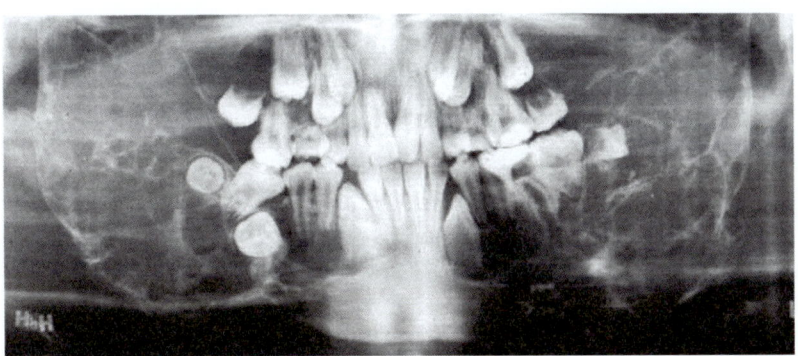

Fig. 65.3.

66. Emphysema subcutaneum iatrogenica

With compressed air input against an open root canal air may be allowed to accumulate in the connective tissue and subcutis. On palpation the tissue "crackles" like crackling parchment. The air disappears within a few days without treatment, but prophylactic antibiotics should be given. Fig.66.1.

67. Epstein's pearls

Small keratin cysts in the palate in newborns. Do not require treatment. Also called **Bohn's nodules**. One can also find them on the gingiva in newborns. For newborns the name **Gingiva cysts** is preferred. Fig.67.1.

68. Epulis fibromatosum

Common fibroma on the gingiva. Surgically removed. Fig.68.1

69. Epulis gravidarum

Also known as pregnancy tumour or granuloma gravidarum. Histopathologically identical to a pyogenic granuloma. Removed surgically after the birth because relapse is high during pregnancy. Fig.69.1.

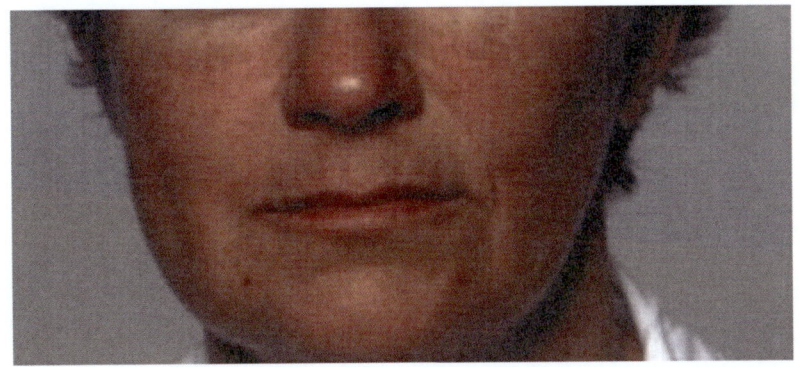

Fig. 66.1.

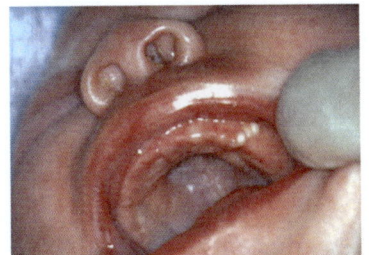

Fig. 67.1.

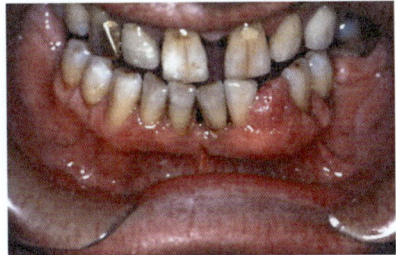

Fig. 68.1.

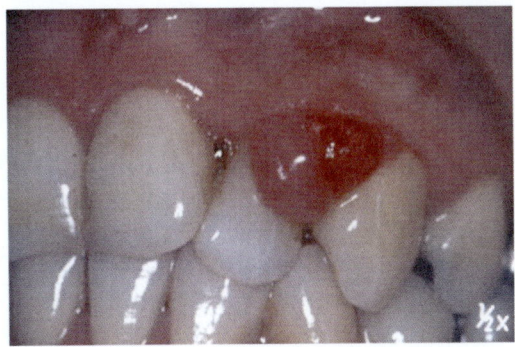

Fig. 69.1.

70. Erythema multiforme exudativum

Definition: Symptom complex with involvement of the skin and mucous membrane.

Aetiology: Can be triggered by medicines, infections, endocrine changes and immunological disorders.

Symptoms: Ulceration, discomfort when swallowing.

Clinical features: Affects mainly young people between 20 and 40 years. Most frequent in men. Naturally lapses in 3-6 weeks. The most severe form is called **Stevens-Johnson syndrome**. It involves ulceration of the mouth, genitalia and eyes as well as fever and malaise, also pharyngitis, arthralgia, myalgia, diarrhoea, etc.. In the mouth there is maculae, later bullae that quickly burst and become erosions, covered with grey-white fibrin and pseudo membranes. The crust formation on the prolabies is very characteristic. Fig.70.1, Fig.70.2 and Fig.70.3.

Diagnosis: Performed on the basis of the clinical profile and medical history. Frequently seen cockade markings in the skin. The histological profile is not pathognomonic for the disorder.

Treatment: Local or systemic steroid. Intravenous fluid therapy. Intraoral antibacterial therapy and local and general pain therapy.

Differential diagnosis: Herpetic gingivostomatitis. Pemphigoid. Pemphigus. Erosive Lichen planus. Stomatitis aftosa recurrens.

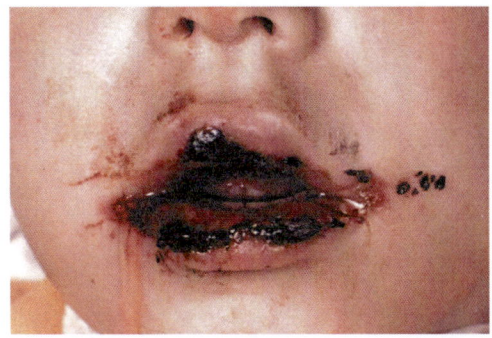

Fig. 70.1.

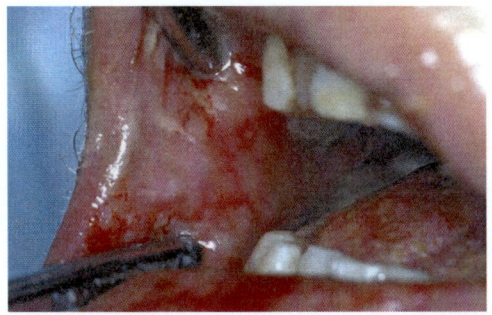

Fig. 70.2.

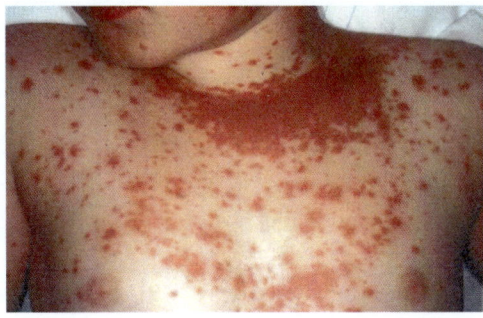

Fig. 70.3.

71. Erythroplakia mucosae oris

Definition: A red change which cannot be diagnosed as any other known disease.

Aetiology: Unknown.

Symptoms: None.

Clinical features: A bright red, often well-defined area, sometimes with a velvety surface Fig.71.1, Fig.71.2 and Fig.71.3.

Diagnosis: Performed clinically and by biopsy. It is a clinical diagnosis of exclusion.

Treatment: Biopsy, excision. Histological examination. Histopathologically it is often a serious diagnosis, i.e. severe epithelial carcinoma in situ or carcinoma.

Differential diagnosis: Atrophic lichen. Benign mucous membrane pemphigoid.

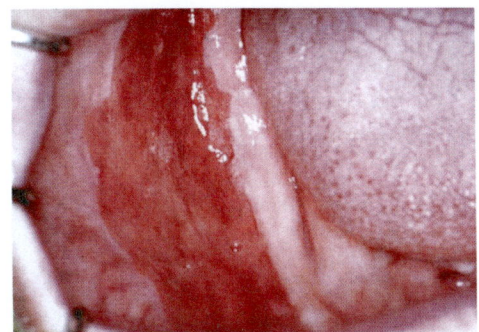

Fig. 71.1.

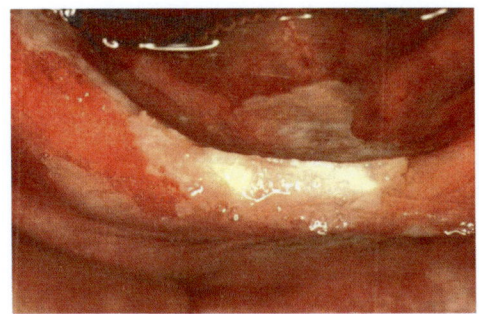

Fig. 71.2.

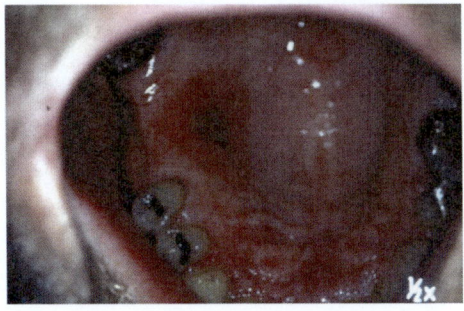

Fig. 71.3.

145

72. Fibroma

Definition: A benign connective tissue tumor.

Aetiology: The cause is unknown. Genuine tumors are relatively rare in the mouth. Most "fibromas" in the mouth are reactive hyperplasias (irritation hyperplasias) which have emerged as a response to a local trauma or irritation. If these are included, the condition is frequent.

Symptoms: Asymptomatic swelling of the mucous membrane.

Clinical features: Can occur anywhere in the mouth but is most often seen in cheek mucous membrane. It presents as a tumour-like asymptomatic swelling with a smooth surface, and with the same colour as the surrounding mucous membrane. It can be stalked or broad-based attached to the mucous membrane Fig.72.1 and Fig.72.2. Most common in the 40-60 age range. Sometimes there is frictional hyperkeratinization on the surface.

Irritation fibromas are most often seen along the bite plane in the cheek, Fig.72.3., and lower lip.

Diagnosis: Performed clinically and by biopsy.

Treatment: Surgical excision. Recurrence very rare.

Differential diagnosis: Lipoma. Pleomorph adenoma. Fibroblastic granuloma with ossification.

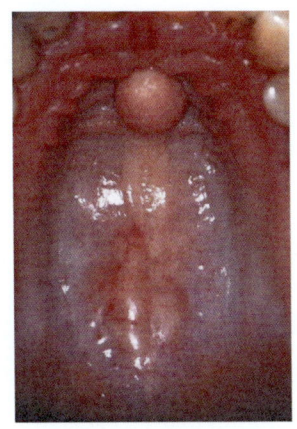

Fig. 72.1.

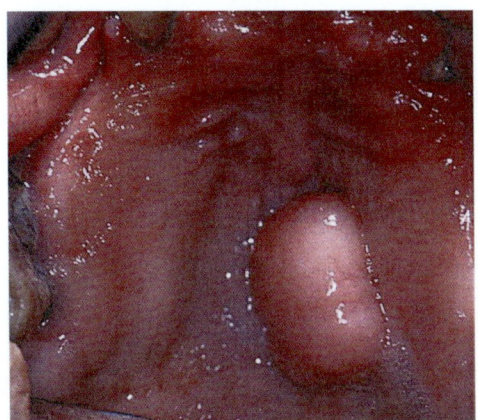

Fig. 72.2.

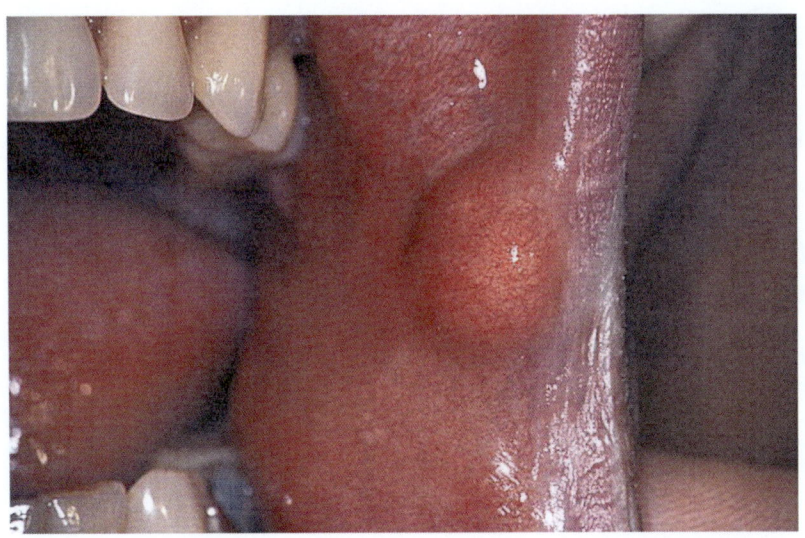

Fig. 72.3.

73. Fibromatosis gingivae

Definition: Isolated gingival enlargement caused by collagen growth in the connective tissue.

Aetiology: Hereditary, autosomal dominant or idiopathic.

Symptoms: None or bad breath and mechanical irritation.

Clinical features: Equal distribution between men and women. Often starts before 15 years old. Most frequent in the maxilla. Gums are firm, fibrous, most often it is generalised, but may be localised to only one quadrant or the molars. Fig.73.1, Fig.73.2 and Fig.73.3.

Diagnosis: Performed on the medical history and clinic and possibly a histological examination.

Treatment: Surgical removal. High recurrence rate. Optimum hygiene.

Differential diagnosis: Medication-induced hyperplasia. General disorders (syndromes).

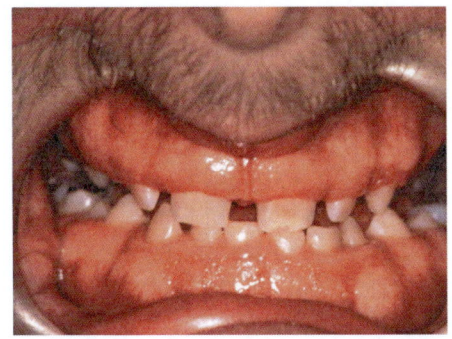

Fig. 73.1.

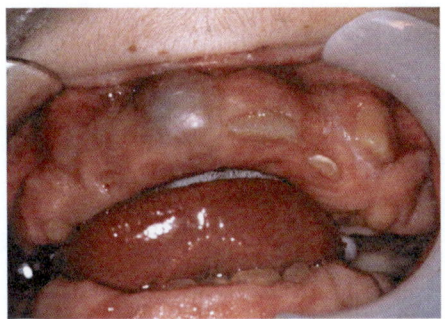

Fig. 73.2.

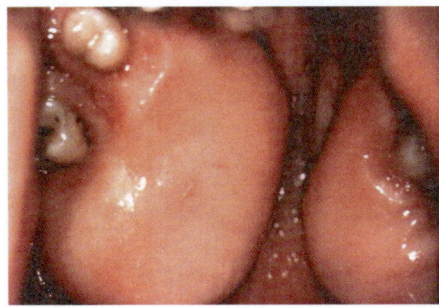

Fig. 73.3.

74. Fibrosarcoma

Definition: Malignant soft tissue tumour originating from the mesenchymal tissue.

Aetiology: Unknown.

Symptoms: Swelling, pain and loosening of teeth.

Clinical features: Most commonly seen in children and adolescents. Most often localised to the gingiva, Fig.74.1, cheek, palate, tongue and lips. X-rays often show teeth without bone surround, Fig.74.2.

Diagnosis: Performed by biopsy and histological examination.

Treatment: Resection, reference to a specialist unit.

Differential diagnosis: Fibroblastic granuloma with ossification. Other malignant mesenchymal tumours.

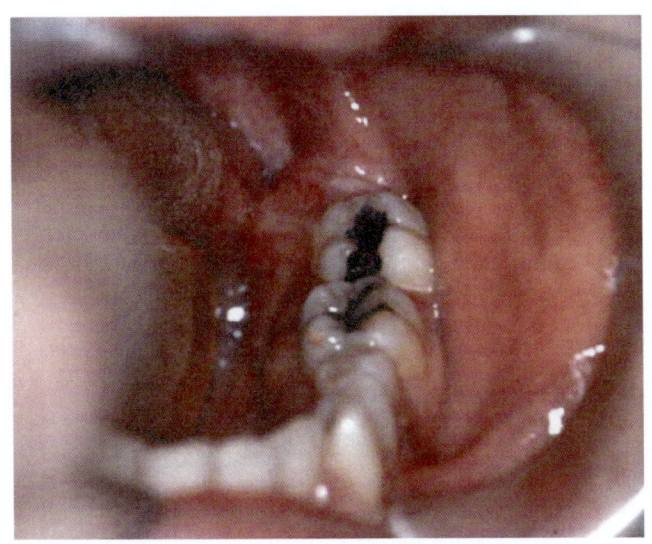

Fig. 74.1.

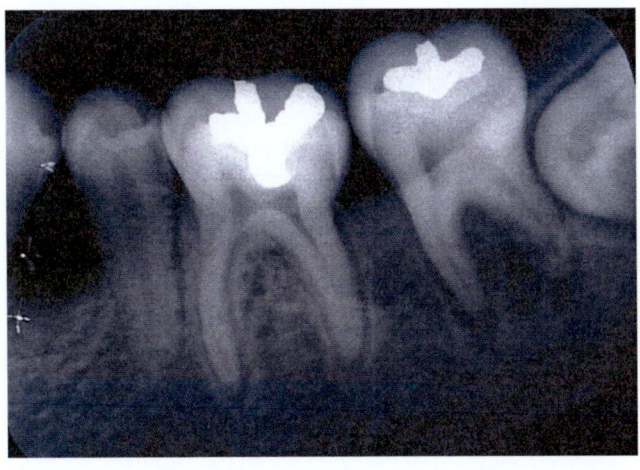

Fig. 74.2.

151

75. Fistula

Definition: A pathologically formed epithelial lined pipe that connects an inflammatory process and a surface.

Aetiology: A fistula occurs when an inflammatory process moves to the skin (**Fistula cutis**) or to the mucous membrane (**Fistula mucosae oris**) to create the drain.

Symptoms: Flow of pus. The pain will ease when the fistula is established. Many patients have chronic fistulas for years.

Clinical features: A fistula in the face or in the mouth will always be preceded by a period of pain and swelling (abscess), Fig.75.1, Fig.75.2. Clinically, it will be possible to express the pus from the area. A fistula can also be established from the maxillary sinus to the oral cavity Fig.75.3 or from the nasal cavity to the oral cavity.

Diagnosis: Performed clinically, possibly with a small scale which can be inserted into the fistula at the point of treatment.

Treatment: The fistula is not treated per se, but it is necessary to treat the cause of the fistula.

Differential diagnosis: None.

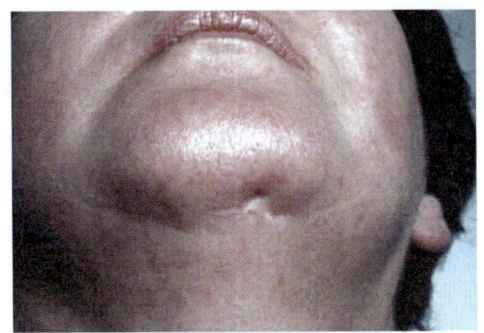

Fig. 75.1.

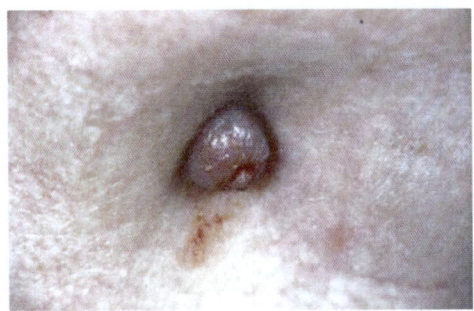

Fig. 75.2.

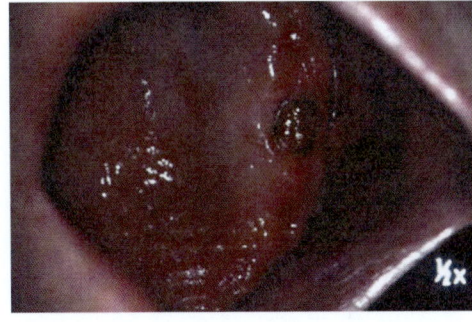

Fig. 75.3.

153

76. Fordyce's spots

Definition: Sebaceous glands scattered in the oral mucous membrane.

Symptoms: The condition is asymptomatic, normal anatomical structure, individual patients feel roughness.

Clinical features: Fordyce spots or granules appear as yellow or yellow-white bumps that commonly occur in clusters on the buccal mucous membrane or laterally on the upper lip prolabium. They are most commonly seen in adults, presumably as a result of hormonal factors, since it is known that puberty stimulates the development of these. There is great variation in the pattern of manifestation, some have only a few granules, while others may have hundreds of them, Fig.76.1, Fig.76.2.

Diagnosis: Performed clinically and by biopsy.

Treatment: None, since the condition is a normal anatomic variation.

Differential diagnosis: Tumour. Mucous membrane cysts.

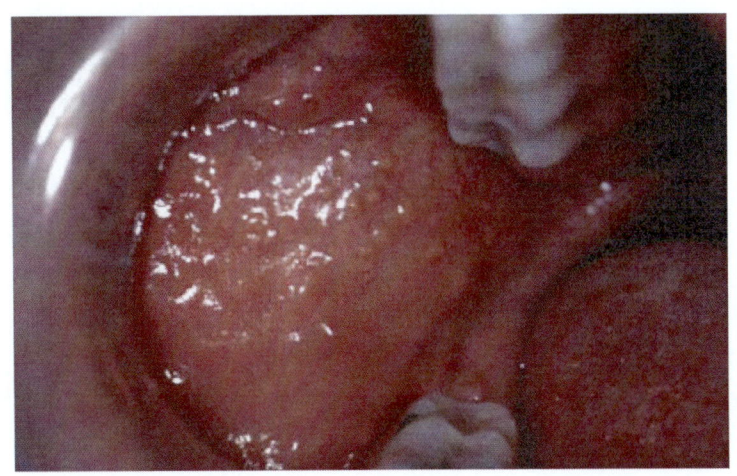

Fig. 76.1.

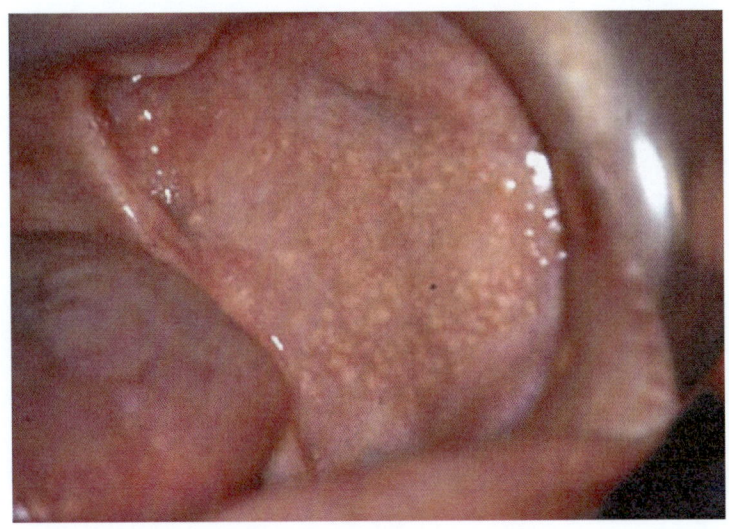

Fig. 76.2.

77. Frenulum anomale labii superioris

Definition: Abnormally short ligament that causes functional problems.

Aetiology: Congenital, and may occur after trauma and subsequent scarring.

Symptoms: Difficulty in moving the lip and pain on activity. Diastema mediale.

Clinical features: When the lip is activated passively an anaemic area corresponding to the papilla incisiva can be seen. Fig.77.1.

Diagnosis: Performed from the medical history and clinical findings.

Treatment: Surgical removal. Must be performed on the palatal side.

Differential diagnosis: None.

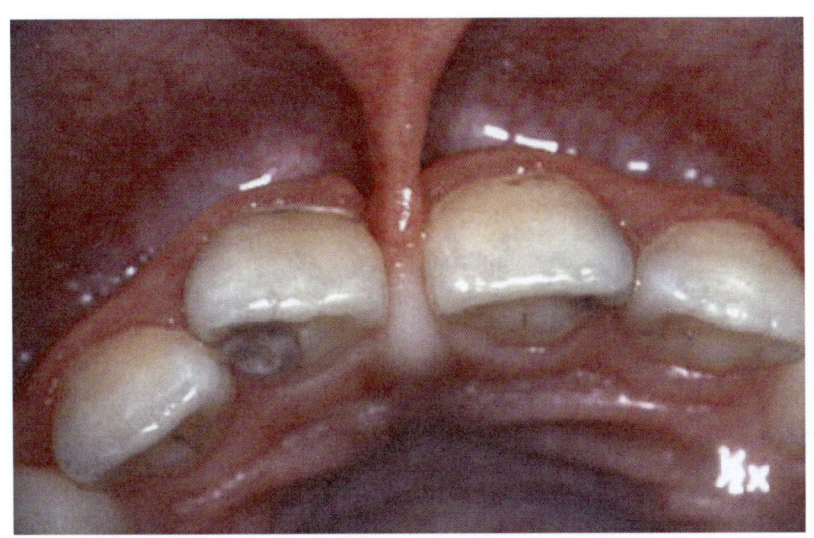

Fig. 77.1.

78. Frenulum anomale linguae

Definition: The ligament is too short when there are functional problems.

Aetiology: Congenital.

Symptoms: Patients frequently complain of finding it difficult to moisten the lips and speak.

Clinical features: The tongue curls with the tip down while attempting to roll the tongue out. There can also be speaking and swallowing problems. Fig.78.1 and Fig.78.2.

Diagnosis: Performed clinically and by medical history.

Treatment: Surgical removal of the ligament.

Differential diagnosis: None.

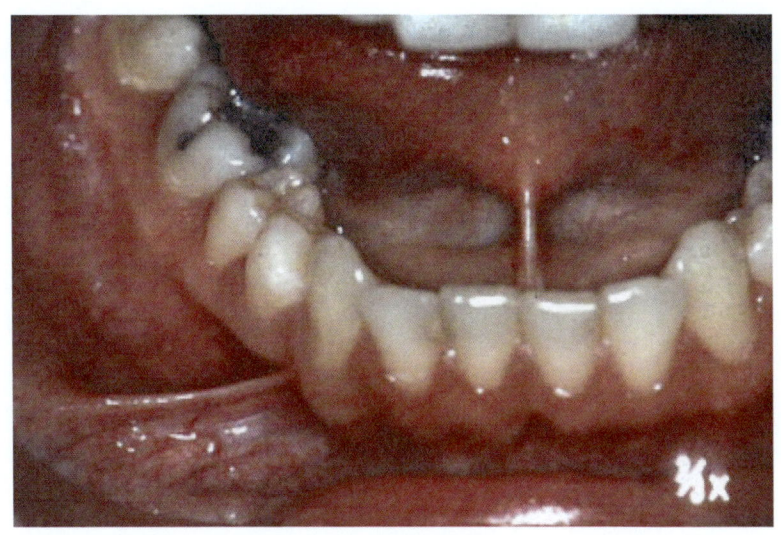

Fig.78.1.

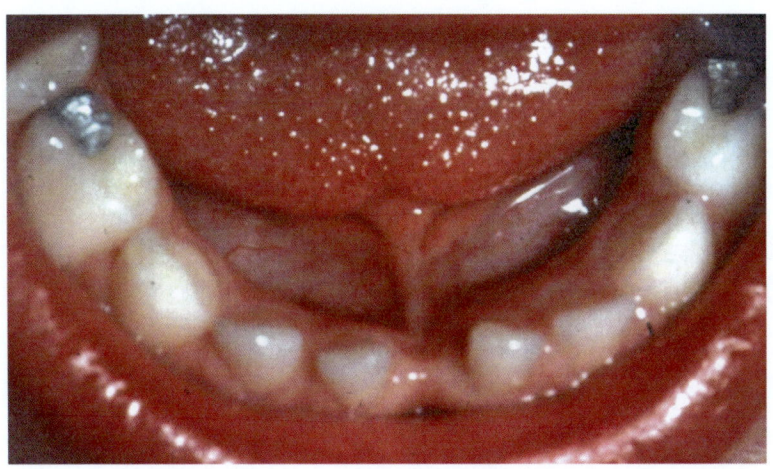

Fig.78.2.

79. Gingivitis

Definition: An inflammatory reaction in the gingiva caused by bacterial deposits, plaque.

Aetiology: The soft bacterial deposits on the teeth. Bacterial toxins and metabolic products lead to an inflammatory response in the marginal gingiva. This is a reversible condition which can be normalised if the bacterial coatings are removed and prevented from re-emerging. Smoking, oral breathing, stress, malnutrition and diabetes mellitus are other factors that produce more gingivitis.

Symptoms: There are few subjective symptoms. The gums bleed when brushing

Clinical features: The gingiva are swollen, red and glossy with loss of normal chagrining, there is bleeding on probing in the pockets. Fig.79.1. If the patient is pregnant the disorder is termed: gingivitis gravidarum, Fig.79.2.

Diagnosis: Performed clinically, bleeding by probing.

Treatment: Instrumental removal of the bacterial coatings (teeth cleaning). In the acute phase this can be supported by rinsing with chlorhexidine 0.1% or brushing with chlorhexidine gel. Patient instruction in proper oral hygiene.

Differential diagnosis: Herpetic gingivostomatitis. Leukaemia. Atrophic lichen planus. Pemphigoid.

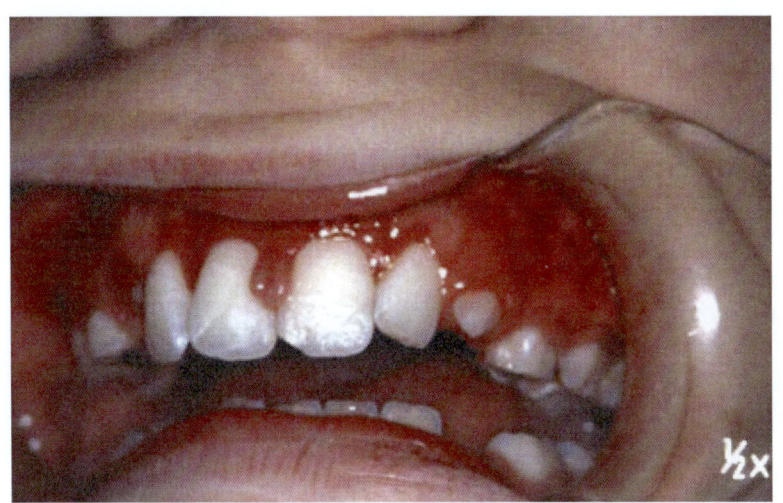

Fig. 79.1.

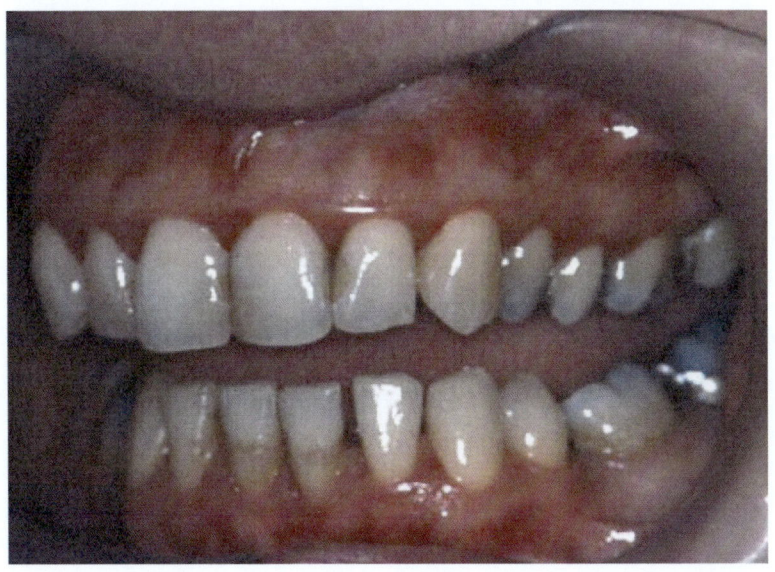

Fig. 79.2.

161

80. Gingivitis hyperplastica

Definition: Hyperplasia of the marginal gingiva.

Aetiology: Idiopathic, pharmacological. In particular, treatment with anti-epileptic agents, Diphydan, Cyclosporin.

Symptoms: Slow growing gingiva.

Clinical features: Characteristic hyperplasias, especially in the papillae. Fig.80.1, Fig.80.2 and Fig.80.3

Diagnosis: Performed clinically and from the medical history.

Treatment: Surgical removal. Large tendency to relapse.

Differential diagnosis: Fibromatosis gingivae. Periodontitis. Leukaemia, Wegener's granulomatosis.

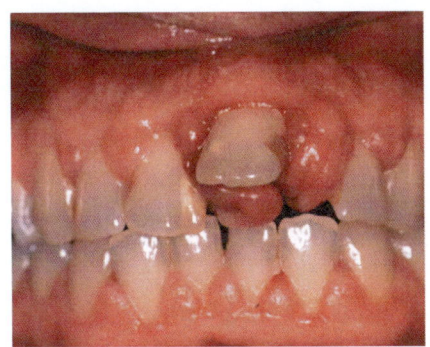

Fig. 80.1.

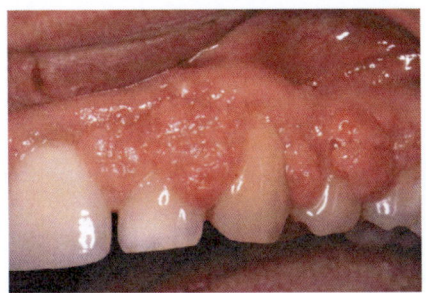

Fig. 80.2.

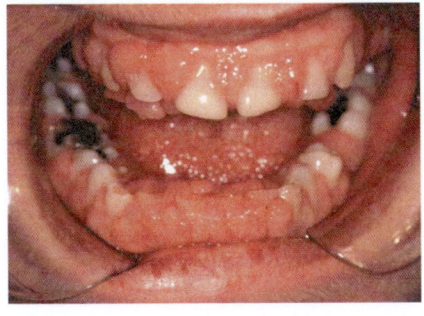

Fig. 80.3.

81. Gingivitis nekroticans

Definition: Gingivitis marked by deep necrosis.

Aetiology: Special gram-negative bacterial flora fusobacteria, spiriller and spirochetes.

Symptoms: Very prutrid odour from the mouth. Pain and bleeding from the gums.

Clinical features: The smell is unmistakable. Large interdental necrosis. Had almost disappeared, but reappeared in highly compromised patients such as persons with HIV and AIDS infection, Fig. 81.1 and Fig. 81.2.

Diagnosis: Performed clinically and from the medical history. Bacterial testing can also help.

Treatment: Antibiotics, Chlorhexidine rinsing, H2O2, Scaling.

Differential diagnosis: Agranulocytosis. Leukaemia.

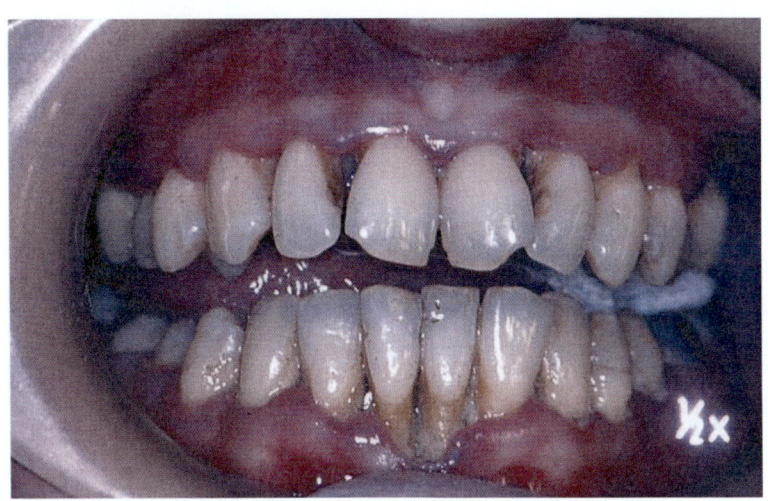

Fig. 81.1.

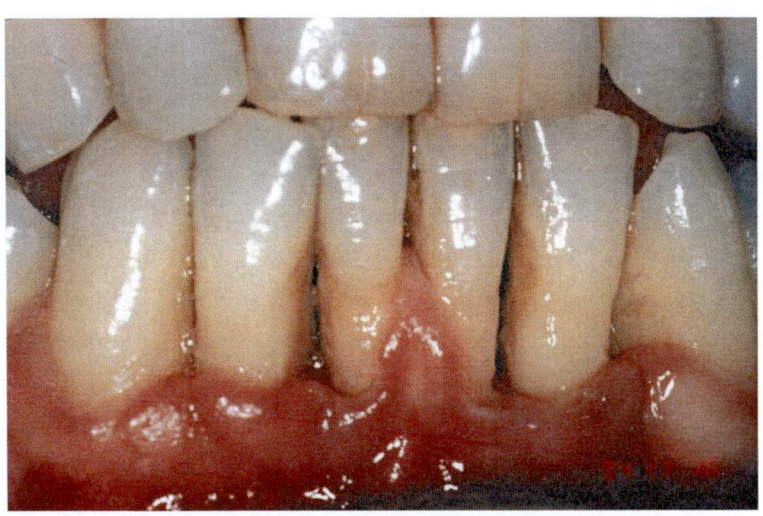

Fig. 81.2.

165

82. Glossitis rhombica mediana

Definition: A benign, reddish change on the dorsum of the tongue in front of the foramen coecum.

Aetiology: There is nearly always a chronic candidiasis - perhaps in a locus minoris resistentiae.

Symptoms: Symptom-free or discomfort when consuming spicy foods.

Clinical features: There is a characteristic rhomboid red area in the middle of the back of the tongue Fig.82.1 and Fig.82.2. The surface can range from smooth to lobular, sometimes hardened. Exclusively in adults.

Diagnosis: Performed clinically, smear.

Treatment: Antifungal therapy. Large tendency to relapse. Tongue hygiene.

Differential diagnosis: Lingua geographica. Carcinoma.

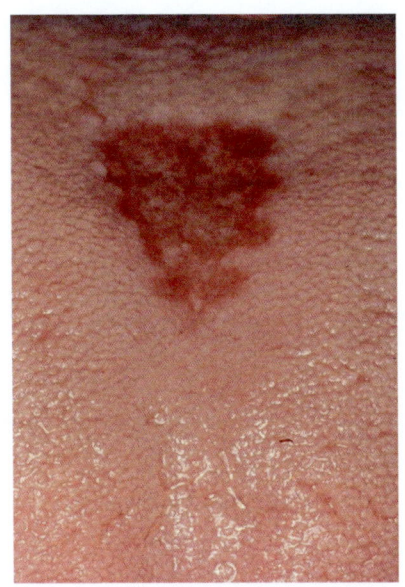

Fig. 82.1.

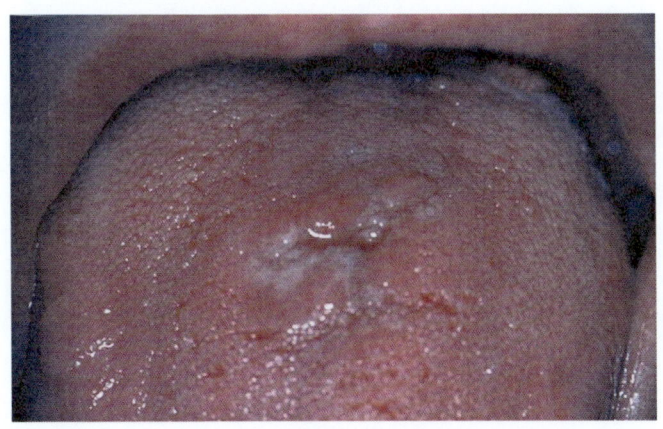

Fig. 82.2.

83. Gorlins syndrome

Definition: Also called basal cell carcinoma syndrome. A complex of several common clinical features.

Aetiology: Unknown.

Symptoms: Symptoms may vary depending on the dominant part of the disorder.

Clinical features: In addition to the basal cell carcinoma that are keratocysts, calcification of the falx cerebri, bifide ribs, increased tendency to brain tumours and intracranial calcifications. Fig.83.1, Fig.83.2 and Fig.83.3.

Diagnosis: Clinical, by combining the various elements.

Treatment: There is no curative treatment, but the individual elements must be treated as needed.

Differential diagnosis: Keratocyst.

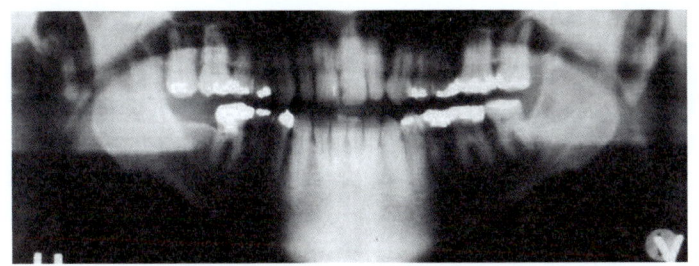

Fig. 83.1.

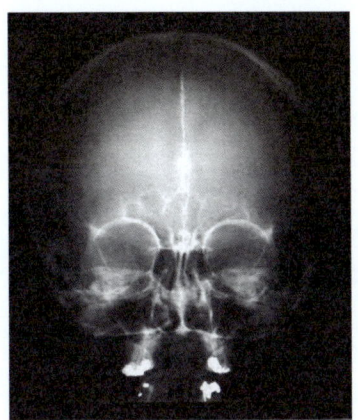

Fig. 83.2.

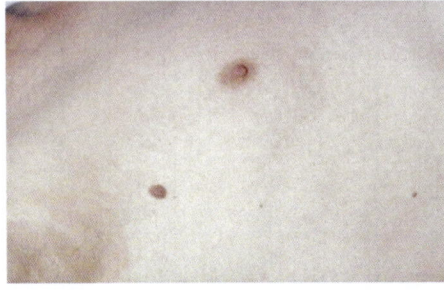

Fig. 83.3.

169

84. Granuloma pyogenicum

Definition: Pyogenic granuloma which is a tumour-like overgrowth of granulation tissue.

Aetiology: Caused by a local irritant agent or trauma.

Symptoms: Asymptomatic, red swelling.

Clinical features: Seen most commonly in children and adolescents. More frequent in women than in men. Appearing as an exophytic, tumour-like mass that can be stemmed or broad-based attached to the underlying tissue. The surface is smooth or lobulated and sometimes ulcerated. It is red to bluish colour, and the size varies between 5 and 10 mm. About 75% is localised to the gingiva, more often in the maxilla than the mandible. Other, but less frequent locations are the lip, the tongue or the buccal mucosa, Fig.84.1, Fig.84.2. In pregnancy the so-called "epulis gravidarum", Fig.84.3 or granuloma gravidarum can be seen. This is due to increased levels of oestrogen and progesterone, in particular in months 3 and 8 of pregnancy.

Diagnosis: Performed clinically and by biopsy.

Treatment: PG must be surgically removed. Preguancy epulis will often undergo spontaneous recovery after the birth. Otherwise, it must be surgically removed.

Differential diagnosis: Peripheral giant cell granuloma. Fibroblastic granuloma with ossification. Metastasis. Kaposi's sarcoma.

170

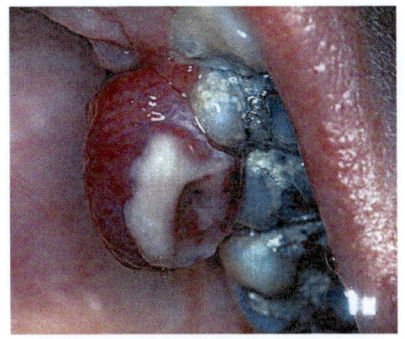

Fig. 84.1.

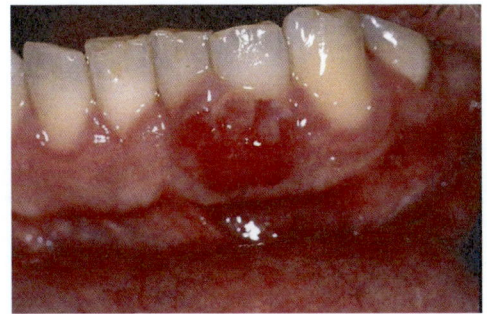

Fig. 84.2.

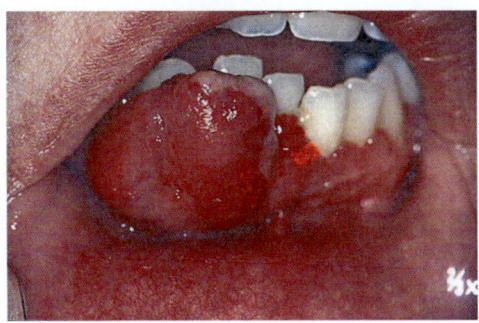

Fig. 84.3.

171

85. Haemangioma

Definition: Benign proliferation of blood vessels.

Aetiology: Unknown.

Symptoms: No, cosmetic nuisance.

Clinical features: There are 3 types: arterial, venous and arterio-venous angiomas. The one with bluish discoloration is located near the surface. Those that lies deep in the connective tissue have a less noticeable colour. Attacks both skin and mucosal membrane. If an intraoral hemangioma is located in an area of operations, it is recommended to refer to a specialist department. Fig.85.1, Fig.85.2 and Fig.85.3.

Diagnosis: performed by means of a slide, in which the lesion can be "blanched".

Treatment: Cryotherapy by small lesions, laser therapy, embolization or general steroid therapy. Also injection of sclerosing agents performed in a specialised unit.

Differential diagnosis: Lymphangioma. Naevus.

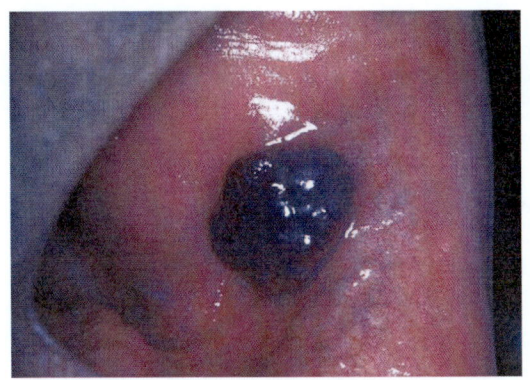

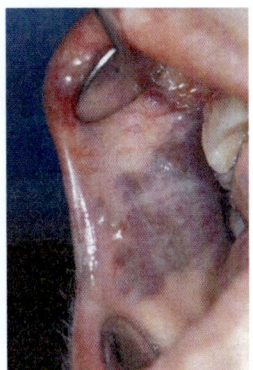

Fig. 85.1.   Fig. 85.2

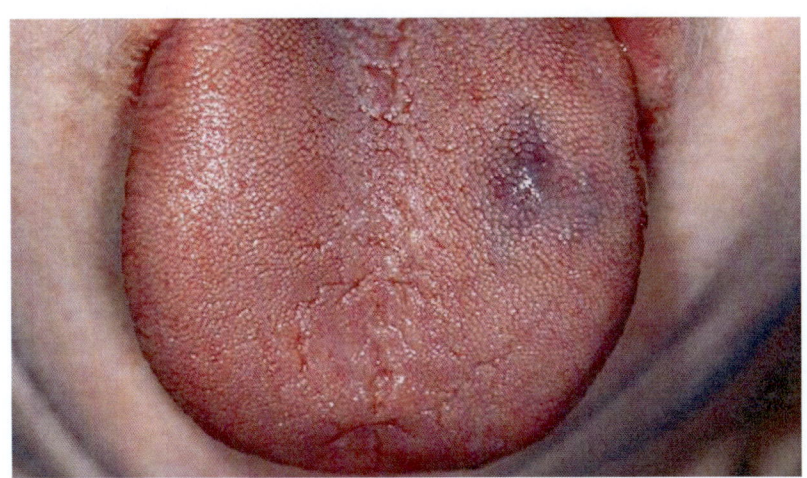

Fig. 85.3.

86. Haematoma

Definition: Accumulation of blood outside the vascular bed.

Aetiology: Lesion of a vessel.

Symptoms: Swelling and pain, as well as multiple colours.

Clinical features: Most often seen after surgery. Lesion of a vessel without adequate haemostasis. Can also be seen in patients in anticoagulant therapy as well as with unknown haemorrhagic diathesis. With unexpected and abnormal bleeding, it should be tested for, Fig.86.1. Fig.86.2 and Fig.86.3 show quite abnormal bleeding and haematoma after oral surgery. In both cases, the cause was an undiagnosed blood disease. Disappears over 2-3 weeks and ends with "multiple" colours in the skin.

Diagnosis: Performed from the medical history.

Treatment: None. After a few days, the settlement is accelerated by heat treatment of the area. As a prophylactic penicillin is administered, as there can easily be infection in a haematoma.

Differential diagnosis: Abscess.

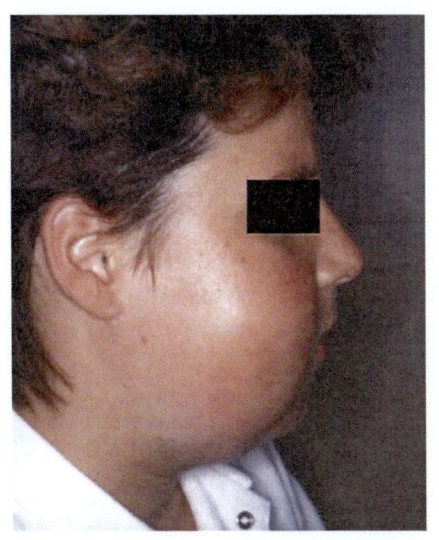

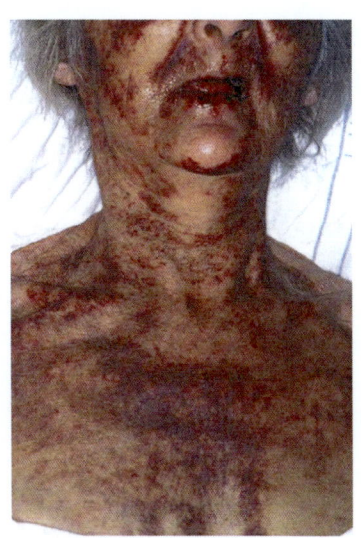

Fig. 86.1.   Fig. 86.2.

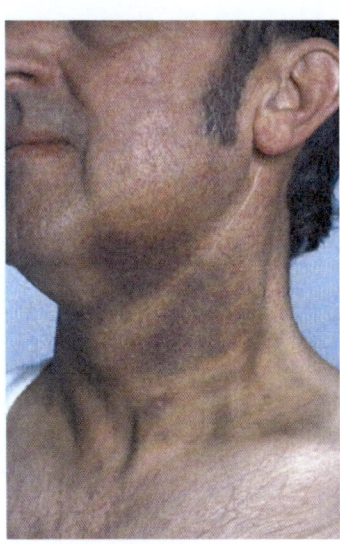

Fig. 86.3.

87. Hairy tongue

Definition: A marked accumulation of keratin on the filiform papillae on the dorsum of the tongue, resulting in a hair-like pattern.

Aetiology: Uncertain, but many patients are heavy smokers. Other associated causal factors mentioned: antibiotic therapy, poor oral hygiene, radiation therapy and growth of fungi and bacteria.

Symptoms: Often asymptomatic. Sometimes the patient complains of bad taste and bad breath.

Clinical features: The filiform papillae are long and brown, yellow or black in colour because of the pigment-producing bacteria or staining from tobacco or food. It is localised to the back of the tongue without reaching the tip of the tongue or the side-edges Fig.87.1.

Diagnosis: Performed clinically.

Treatment: Establishing good oral hygiene. Tongue brushing and scraping of the tongue top. A good remedy is to rinse the mouth with a tablespoon of 3% hydrogen peroxide in half a glass of water. 2 times a day.

Differential diagnosis: Candidiasis. Leukoplakia.

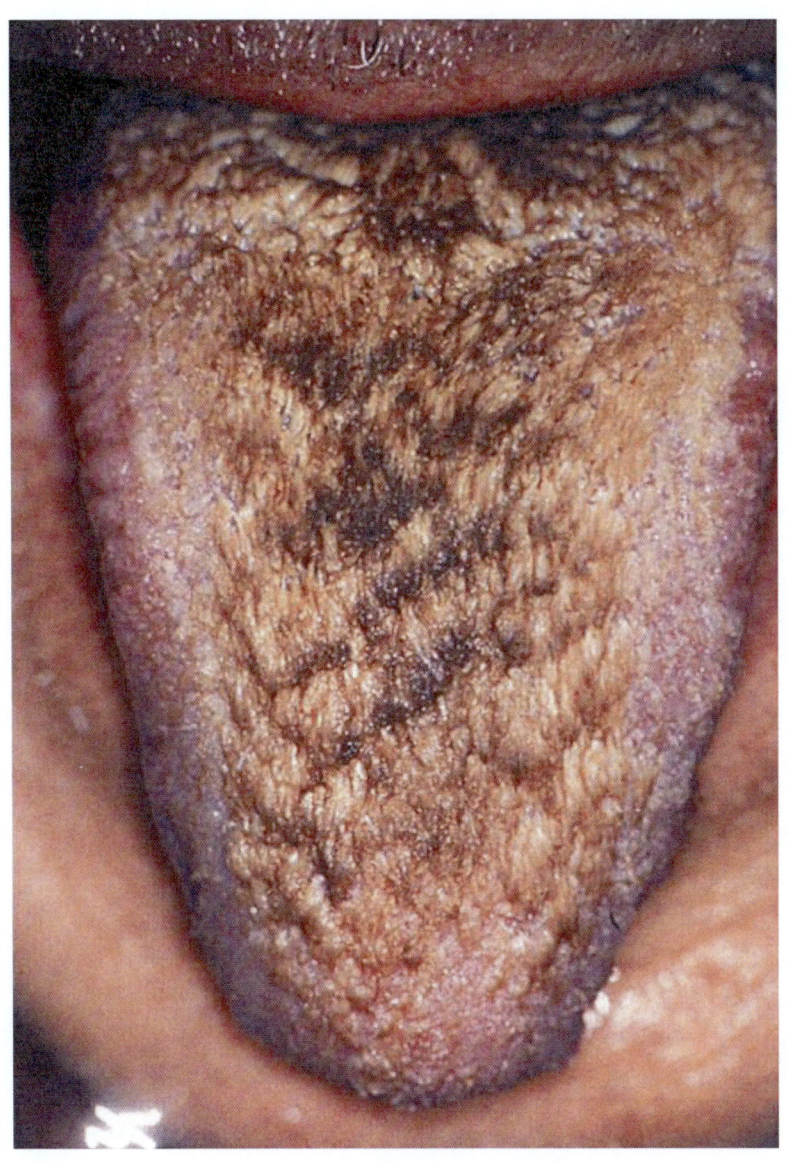

Fig. 87.1.

88. Herpes Zoster

Definition: Reactivation of Varicella-Zoster virus.

Aetiology: Viral infection.

Symptoms: Also called "shingles" because of the almost unbearable pain.

Clinical features: Occurs in all age groups but is most common in the elderly. Frequent in immunocompromised patients. Seen as a hemifacial ulceration, vesicles on a scarlet features. Orally all mucous membranes can be affected. Characterized by great pain. Fig.88.1. Fig.88.2 shows half-sided lesions in the palate.

Diagnosis: Performed on the clinical profile and a blood sample.

Treatment: Acyclovir 800mg 5 time /per day for 5 days starting as early as possible. Complemented by strong analgesic. Vaccination is now an option.

Differential diagnosis: Herpes simplex, Erythema multiforme.

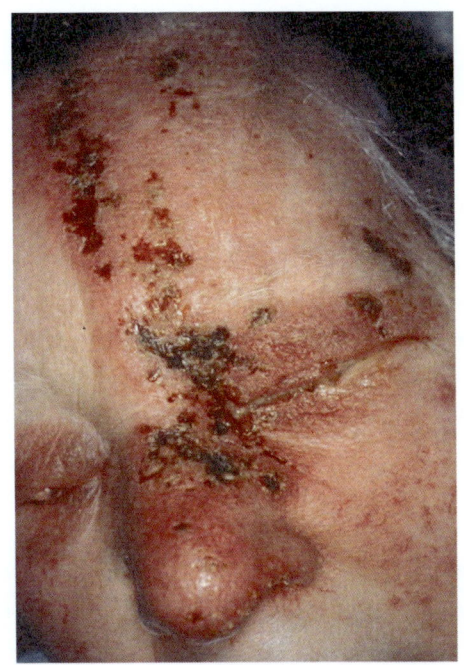

Fig. 88.1.

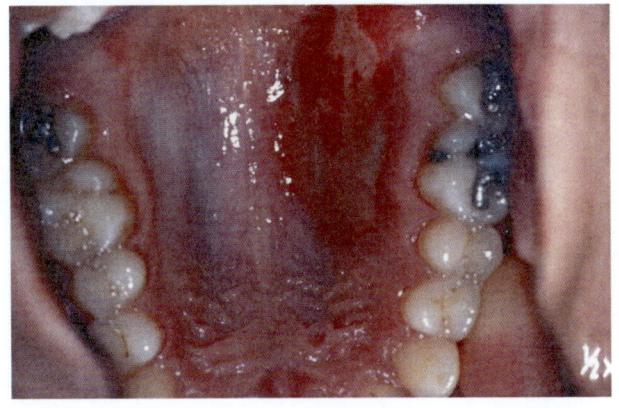

Fig. 88.2.

179

89. Herpetic gingivostomatitis, herpes labialis

Definition: Oral infection with the herpes simplex virus (HSV).

Aetiology: In 90% of cases the infection is caused by HSV type 1.

Symptoms: Fever, pain and swelling lymph nodes.

Clinical features: The infection occurs in a primary, acute form, as herpetic gingivostomatitis Fig.89.1 and Fig.89.2, and in a secondary form, as herpes labialis Fig.89.3. The primary infection occurs most frequently in children between ½ to 6 years.

There is an incubation period of 3-9 days. In the mouth, numerous vesicles and ulcers are seen. These will often flow together to form larger eroded areas. The gingiva are raised, bright red and vulnerable. The regional lymph nodes is often swollen and weak. On reactivation, herpes labialis ("cold sores") can be seen. There are small clusters of liquid-filled vesicles, which rupture and leave ulcerations. About 6-24 hours before the outbreak prodromal pain occurs, i.e. an itching or burning sensation in the area.

Diagnosis: The diagnosis is performed on the clinical signs, and by a swab from the vesicles. There may also be a blood test for the clearance of circulating antibodies.

Treatment: Acyclovir.

Differential diagnosis: Aphthous stomatitis. Herpangina. Erythema multiforme.

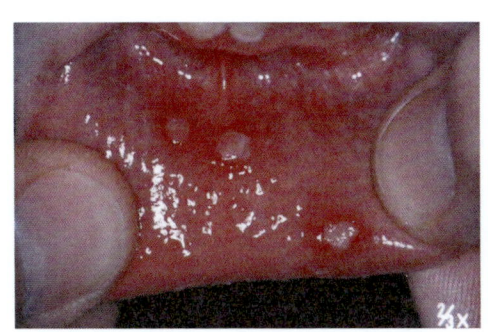

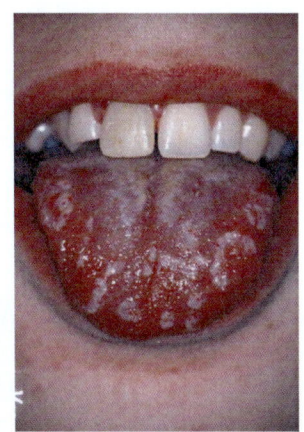

Fig. 89.1.   Fig. 89.2.

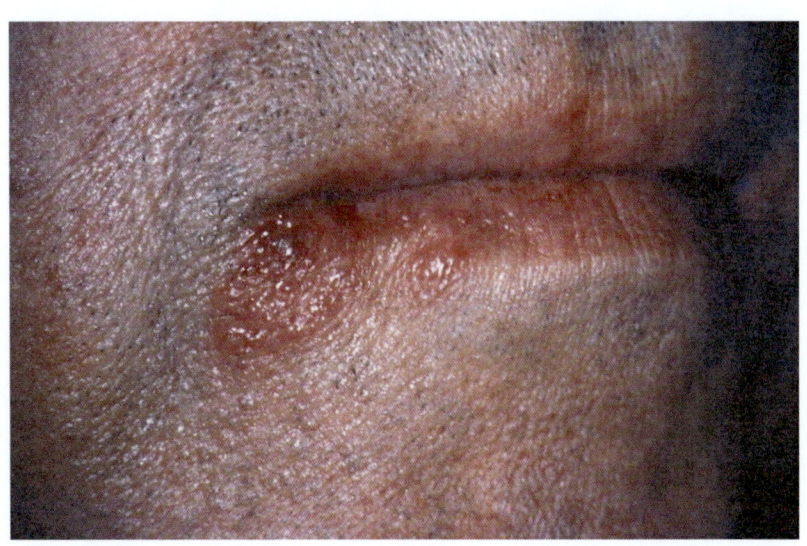

Fig. 89.3.

90. Hyperplasia epitelialis focalis

Definition: Virus-induced, local proliferation of squamous epithelium.

Aetiology: HPV virus, human papillomavirus of type 13 and 32.

Symptoms: No, cosmetic nuisance.

Clinical features: Frequently seen in Eskimos and South Americans, but can also be seen in other peoples. Fig.90.1 and Fig.90.2.

Diagnosis: Performed clinically and histologically.

Treatment: None. Some patients want them removed for aesthetic reasons.

Differential diagnosis: Condyloma acuminatum. Verruca vulgaris. Papilloma.Mb.Crohn.

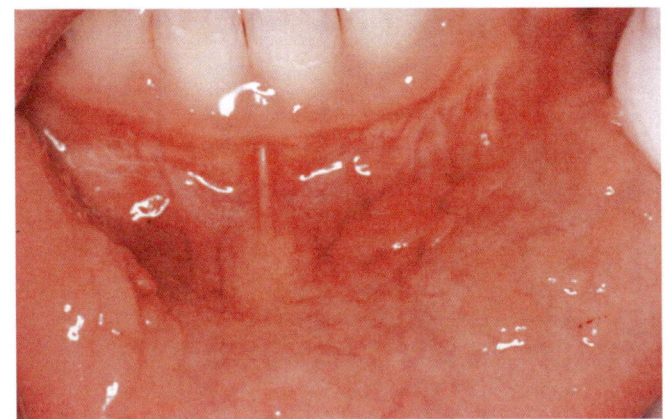

Fig. 90.1.

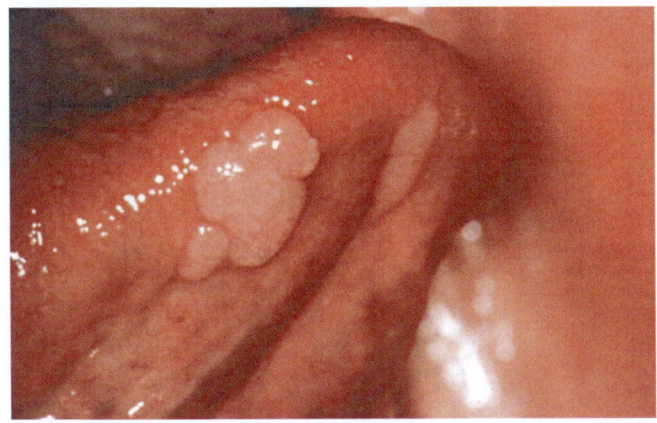

Fig. 90.2.

91. Hyperplasia mucosae oris

Definition: Inflammatory induced hyperplasia of the connective tissue and mucous membrane.

Aetiology: Usually caused by poorly fitting dentures. Irritation hyperplasias or denture curtains.

Symptoms: Inflammation, fungal infections, bad breath and bad denture function.

Clinical features: Most common in denture patients. Fig.91.1, Fig.91.2 and Fig.91.3.

Diagnosis: Performed clinically and possibly histologically.

Treatment: Surgical removal. Fungi treatment. Denture correction.

Differential diagnosis: Carcinoma. Candidosis.

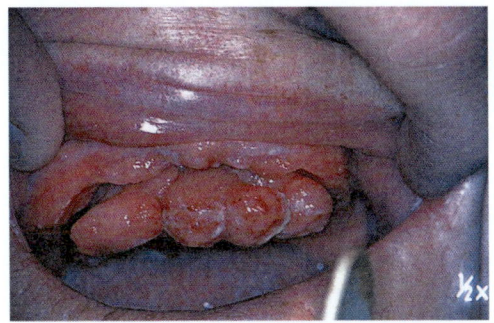

Fig. 91.1.

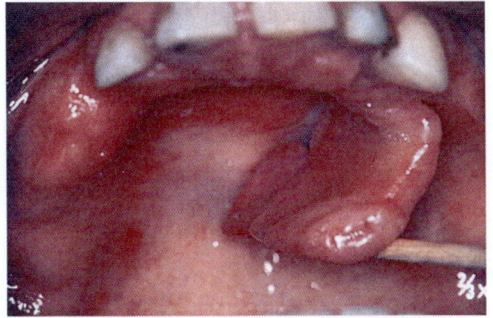

Fig. 91.2.

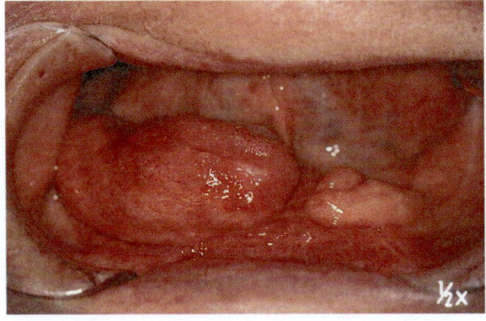

Fig. 91.3.

185

92. Hypertrofia musculus masseterica

Definition: Unilateral enlargement of the individual muscle fibres.

Aetiology: Static hyperactivity.

Symptoms: None.

Clinical features: Slow-growing swelling similar to muscle mass with attachment on mandible. Fig.92.1.

Diagnosis: Performed clinically. Possibly supplemented with ultrasound.

Treatment: Discontinuation of habit. Possibly bite splint. If it is a major cosmetic nuisance, it may be referred to a specialist unit for injection of Botulinum toxin.

Differential diagnosis: None.

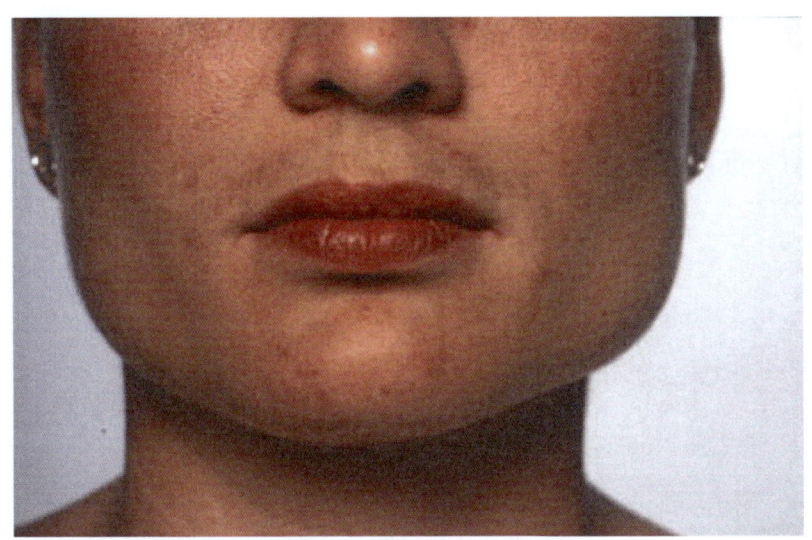

Fig. 92.1.

93. Hypoplasia enameli externa

Definition: Tooth formation disorders presenting as macroscopic defects in the enamel surface.

Aetiology: Systemic defect. Illness, nutritional deficiency or medicine.

Symptoms: Cosmetic discomfort, pain, many dental visits.

Clinical features: Will always affect the same teeth pairs. On the basis of the defect location, it can be calculated when the injury occurred. Loss of biting height. Cosmetic complaints. Large variations in the clinical profile. The prevalence is indicated as between 3-15%. The vast majority of cases are seen in the first 10 months after birth, which involve the first molars and the incisors, except for the lateral ones in the maxilla. Fig.93.1, Fig.93.2 and Fig.93.3.

Diagnosis: Performed clinically.

Treatment: Secure the inter-alveolar distance. Lifelong prevention and dental reconstruction.

Differential diagnosis: Amelogenesis imperfecta. Dentinogenesis imperfecta.

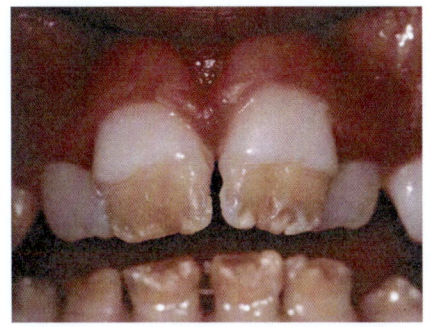

Fig. 93.1.

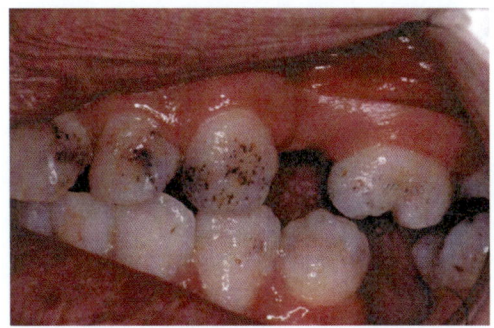

Fig. 93.2.

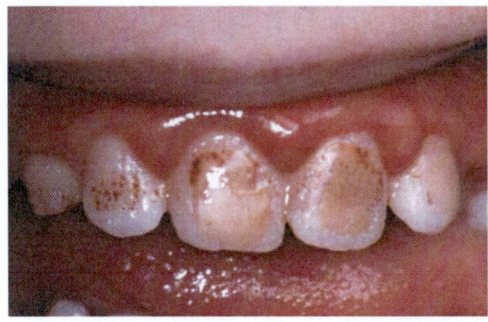

Fig. 93.3.

94. Hypoplasia enameli interna

Definition: Changes in enamel structure but normal surface.

Aetiology: Most frequently trauma on a primary tooth during the formation of the permanent tooth, called **Turner tooth**.

Symptoms: Cosmetic complaints.

Clinical features: Most common in the incisor area. The colour is often yellow to brown. Fig.94.1.

Diagnosis: Performed clinically with a good medical history.

Treatment: Cosmetic treatment.

Differential diagnosis: External enamel hypoplasia.

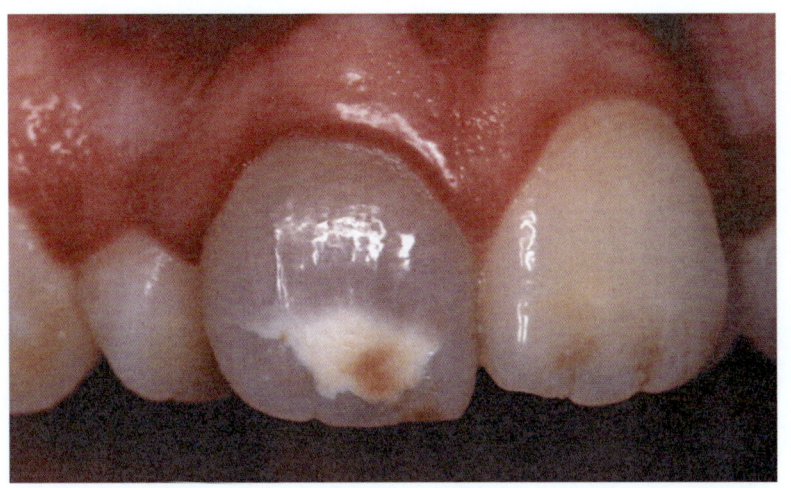

Fig. 94.1

95. Jaw diseases, odontogenic tumours

Odontogenic tumours:

Definition: Tumours developed from the tooth-forming tissue. They are divided into three subgroups based on the presence and distribution of the two neoplastic tissues: odontogenetic epithelium and ectomesencymal tissue. Only selected cases.

Odontoma:

Definition: A tumour in which all the dental tissues are represented, including the hard tissues, enamel and dentine.

The odontoma is the most common odontogenic tumour. It occurs in two kinds: the **composite odontoma**, Fig.95.1.a that resembles a conglomerate of small teeth-like elements Fig.95.1.b, and the **complex**, where the enamel and the dentine is composed in a disorderly pattern. Fig.95.1.c.

Symptoms: No subjective symptoms.

Clinical features: Discovered either as a random radiograph finding or because the tumour has prevented the normal eruption of a tooth. Fig.95.1.d

Diagnosis: By histology and x-rays.

Treatment: Surgical excocleation

Differential diagnosis: Other odontogenic tumours.

192

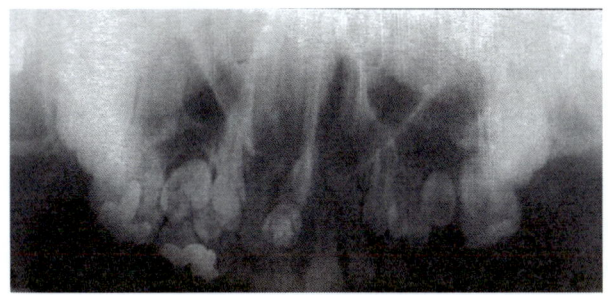

Fig. 95.1.a.

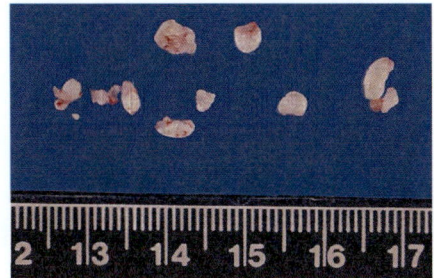

Fig. 95.1.b.

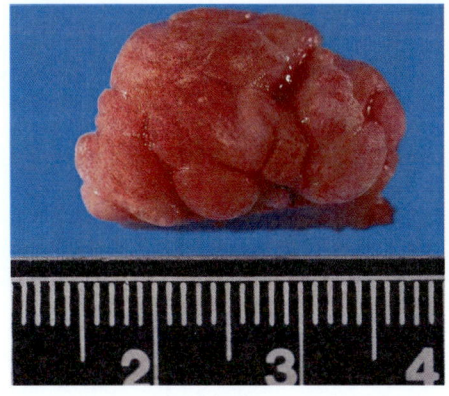

Fig. 95.1.c.

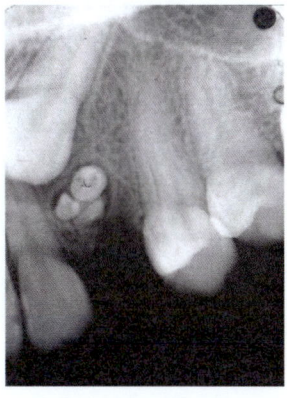

Fig. 95.1.d.

Ameloblastoma

Definition: A benign, locally aggressive tumour consisting of proliferating odontogenetic epithelial tissue.

Aetiology: Unknown.

Symptoms: There is rarely pain, but often swelling in the region.

Clinical features: Most commonly in the 30-40 age range. Most frequently posterior mandibular, Fig.95.2.a and Fig.95.2.b. Can also be seen in the maxilla. Fig.95.2.c shows a scan with the filling of the right maxilla which was histologically shown to be a ameloblastoma.

Diagnosis: Histological.

Treatment: Radical surgery.

Differential diagnosis: Keratocyst. Myxoma. Other odontogenic tumours.

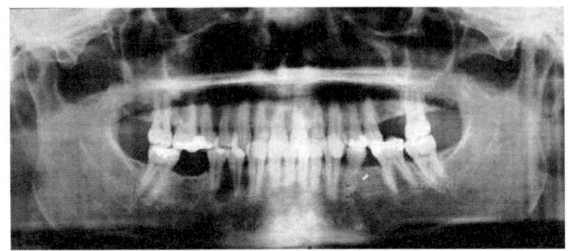

Fig. 95.2.a.

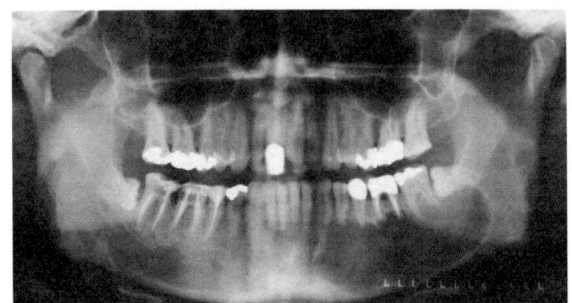

Fig. 95.2.b.

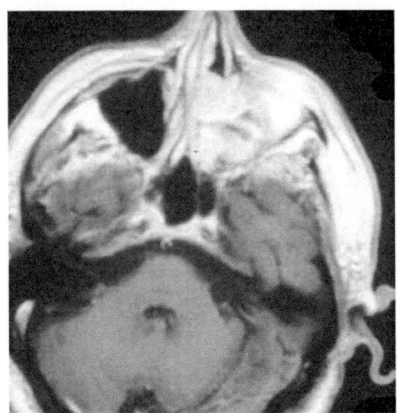

Fig. 95.2.c.

Fibro-osseous jaw diseases

Definition: A group of jaw diseases in which normal bone architecture is replaced by a mesenchymal tissue. This tissue contains a fibrous stroma with fibroblasts and collagen. It also contains varying amounts of mineralized material in the form of a cement-like hard tissue or bone.

There is no question of a specific diagnosis, but a group of several entities, both neoplastic and non-neoplastic. The last group comprises fibrous dysplasia, cemento-osseous dysplasia, aneurysmal bone cyst, central giant cell granuloma and cherubism. The neoplastic conditions are described as cemento-ossifying fibroids. Only the latter will be discussed here.

Cemento-ossifying fibroma:

Definition: Well-defined tumour. Consist of fibrous tissue that contains varying amounts of mineralized material similar to bone and/or cement.

Symptoms: Defiguration of the face.

Clinical features: Little or no pain. Slowly growing swelling of the jaw, Fig.95.3.

Diagnosis: Histological.

Treatment: Surgical removal.

Differential diagnosis: Fibrous dysplasia. Cemento-osseous dysplasias.

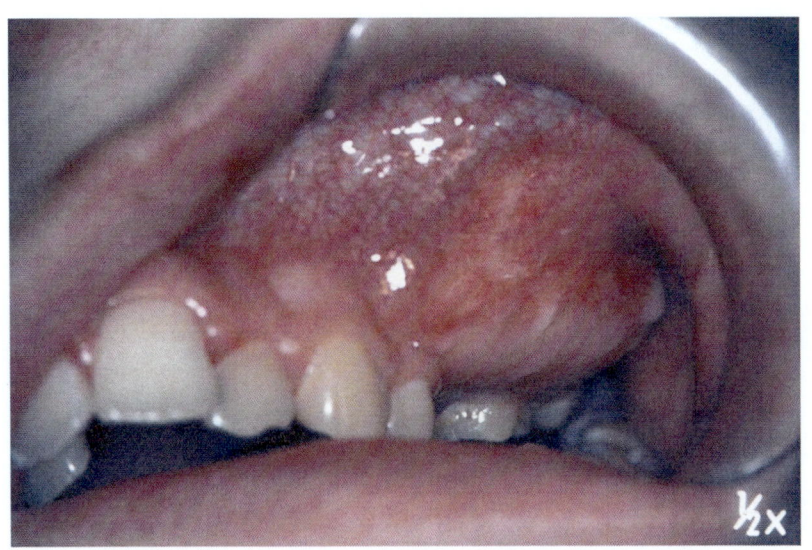

Fig. 95.3.

96. Keratoacantoma

Definition: Benign cutaneous lesion extending from the hair follicles.

Aetiology: Unknown.

Symptoms: None, if any, functional and cosmetic nuisances.

Clinical features: Occurs most frequently on the lips in the 60-70 age range. Slightly raised well-defined lesion with a crater shape centrally and hardened edges, but without evidence of infiltration. Can disappear spontaneously. Fig.96.1.

Diagnosis: Performed by clinical observation, biopsy and histology.

Treatment: Refer to a specialist unit, surgical removal. Recurrence is rare.

Differential diagnosis: Carcinoma. Actinic elastosis.

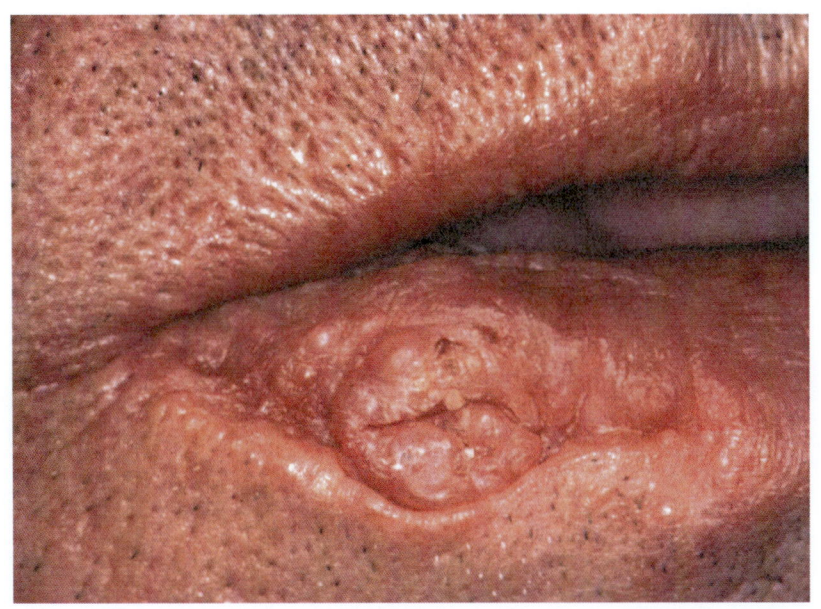

Fig. 96.1.

97. A. Leiomyoma

Definition: Benign tumour originating from the smooth muscle.

Aetiology: Unknown.

Symptoms: Most cases are slow growing and asymptomatic. However, there may be pain.

Clinical features: There are 3 types. Solid, angiomyomer and epithelioid. The colour is normal or bluish. Most frequently seen on the lips, palate, tongue and cheek. Occurs in all ages. Fig.97.1 and Fig.97.2 shows a tumour in a 20 year old woman.

Diagnosis: Performed after biopsy.

Treatment: Surgical removal. Recurrence is rare.

Differential diagnosis: Other tumours. Leiomyosarcoma.

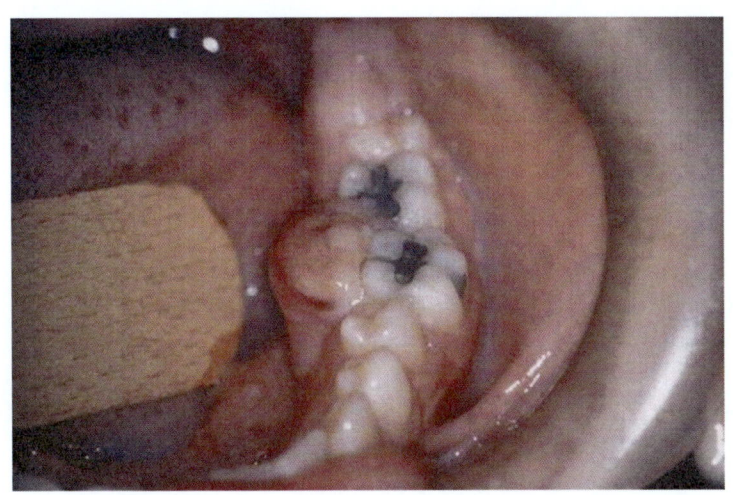

Fig. 97.1.

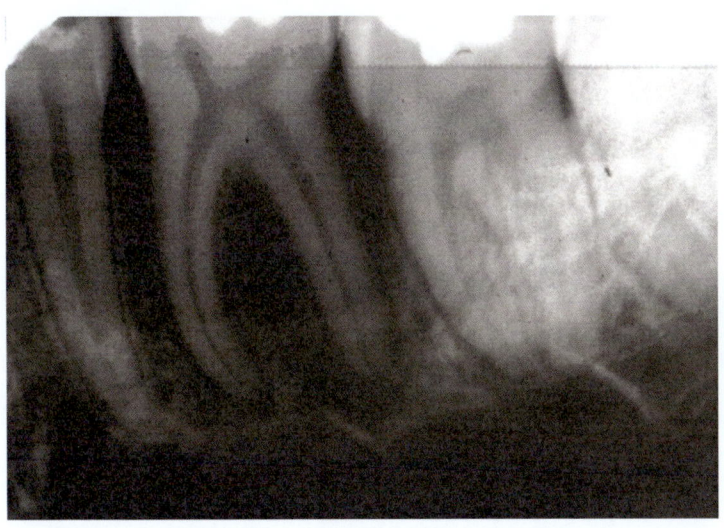

Fig. 97.2.

97. B. Leiomyosarcoma

Definition: Malignant neoplasm of smooth muscle.

Aetiology: Unknown.

Symptoms: None.

Clinical features: Increasing swelling that can ulcerate. Rare in the oral cavity. Most commonly in the middle-aged and older. Fig.97.3.

Diagnosis: Histology.

Treatment: Surgical removal, supported by radiation and chemotherapy. Refer to a specialist unit. The prognosis for oral cases is very bad.

Differential diagnosis: Other tumours - benign and malignant.

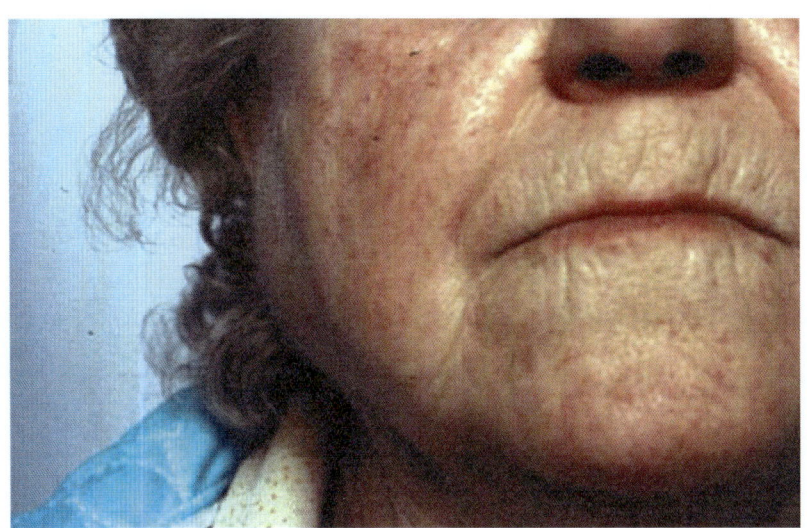

Fig. 97.3.

98. Leukaemia

Definition: Heterogeneous group of malignant diseases of the blood-forming tissues.

Aetiology: Unknown.

Symptoms: Fatigue, weakness, weight loss, fever, headache, pallor, bleeding, infections, bone pain, swollen lymph nodes. Enlarged liver and spleen. Orally ulceration, pain and bleeding will be seen.

Clinical features: The clinical condition will reflect the general symptoms. Ulcerations, bleeding, petechiae, ecchymosis, dental loosening. Swollen gums are an early sign. Fig.98.1. and Fig.98.2.

Diagnosis: Performed on the clinical profile and laboratory tests.

Treatment: Refer to the Oncology Section.

Differential diagnosis: Agranulocytosis, Cyclic neutropenia.

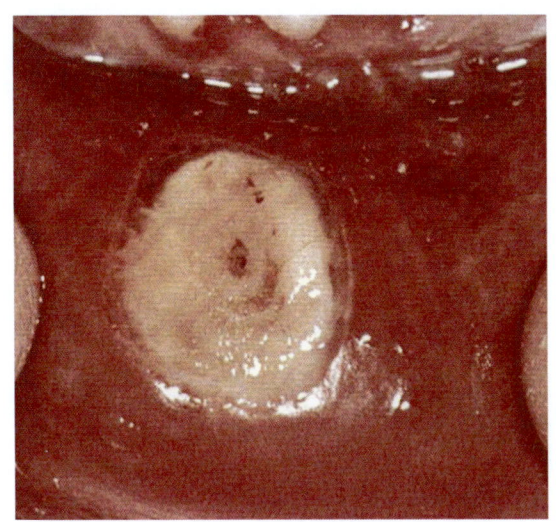

Fig. 98.1.

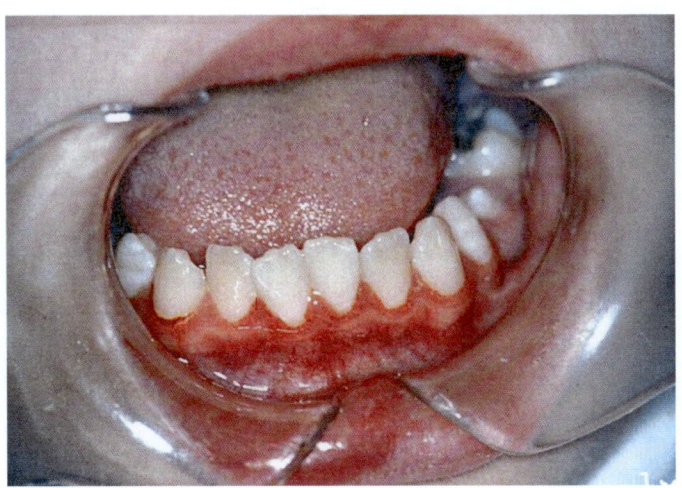

Fig. 98.2.

99. Leukoedema

Definition: A normal anatomic variation in which there is increased thickness of the epithelium and oedema of the epithelium.

Aetiology: Unknown. Perhaps an ethnic predisposition. It is more common in blacks than whites. Also common in smokers.

Symptoms: None

Clinical features: It is characterised by a diffuse, grey-white, milky translucent appearance frequently localised to the buccal mucous membrane bilaterally, Fig.99.1. By stretching the cheek, or by scraping with a spatula it is possible to get the state to almost disappear for a few seconds, after which it returns.

Diagnosis: Performed clinically.

Treatment: None.

Differential diagnosis: Leukoplakia. Candidiasis. Lichen ruber planus.

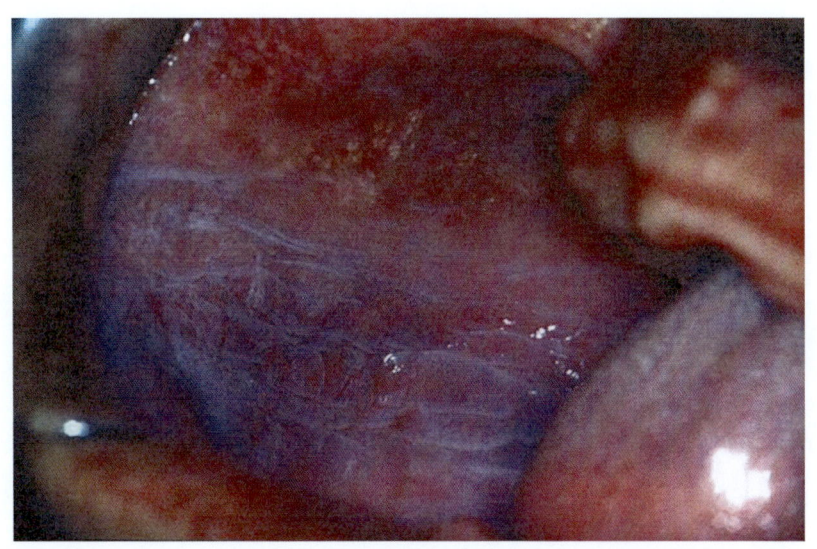

Fig. 99.1.

100. Leukoplakia mucosae oris

Definition: An oral leukoplakia is a predominantly white lesion of the oral mucous membrane and which cannot be diagnosed as any other disease.

This is therefore a **diagnosis of exclusion**. The state is a clinical diagnosis, in which the histopathological profile can range from hyperkeratosis to dysplasias of different levels to invasive carcinoma.

Aetiology: Unknown. However, several factors seem to play a role in the development of leukoplakia and oral cancer. These are tobacco, Candida albicans, and the HPV virus, especially type 18 and 16.

Symptoms: None. Some patients complain of roughness in the mucous membrane.

Clinical features: Leukoplakias are divided into homogenous and non-homogeneous. The latter are sub-divided into erythro-leukoplakias, nodular and exophytic leukoplakia.

A homogeneous leukoplakia is a predominantly white and flat lesion with a uniform appearance. Deep furrows are seen in the cheek and a wavy, puckered surface is seen in the floor of the mouth Fig.100.1, Fig.100.2.

A erythroleukoplakia is a flat lesion consisting of predominantly white and/or red and white changes.

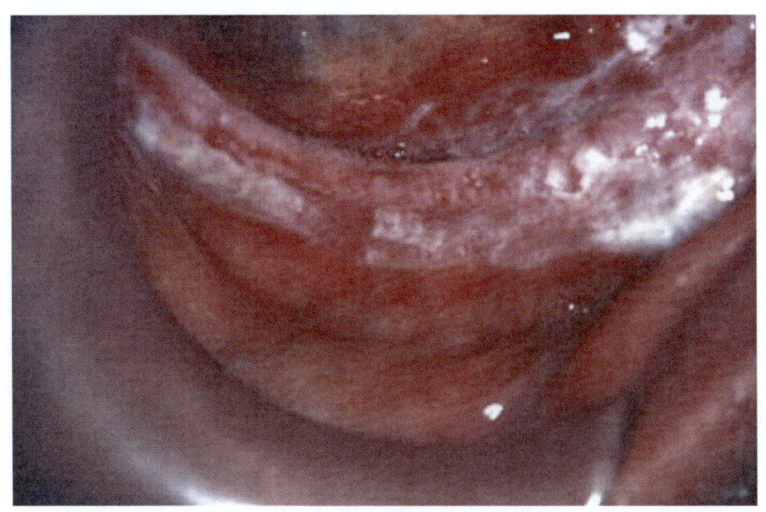

Fig. 100.1.

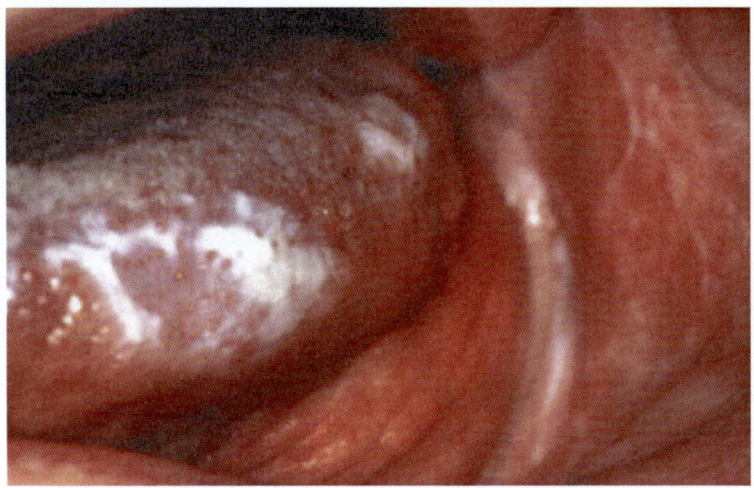

Fig. 100.2.

The nodular leukoplakia has light elevated, roundish white (cotton ball-like) and/or red excrescences. The exophytic are described as thickened leukoplakia with irregular, blunt or sharp projections. There is usually a mixture of different types.

The prevalence in Scandinavia is 3.6% (M: 6.1%; F: 1.2%). The risk of malignant transformation is indicated in Scandinavia to be 5% over 5 years. Non-homogeneous lesions involved, as mentioned, a higher risk of malignant development. Leukoplakias of the bottom of the mouth and the tongue more likely to become malignant. If the patient is non-smoking, yet has a leukoplakia, the risk is greater. All things being equal, women with leukoplakia have greater risk of cancer. If the histological examination shows dysplasia, there is increased risk Fig.100.3 and Fig.100.4.

Treatment: There have over the years been different views on how active it is necessary to be in respect of removing the leukoplakias and in this connection how much the risk of cancer development can be reduced. Today, the practice is generally more active than before, with surgical removal of the leukoplakias. Major research has shown that it is possible to reduce the number of new cancers using the surgical/CO_2 laser to eliminate the lesions. Also, by reducing the etiological factors, such as alkohol, tobacco and candida.

Differential diagnosis: Friction keratosis. Morsicatio. Lichen ruber planus. Discoid LE. Leukokeratosis nicotina palati. Contact lesions. Snuff dippers keratosis.

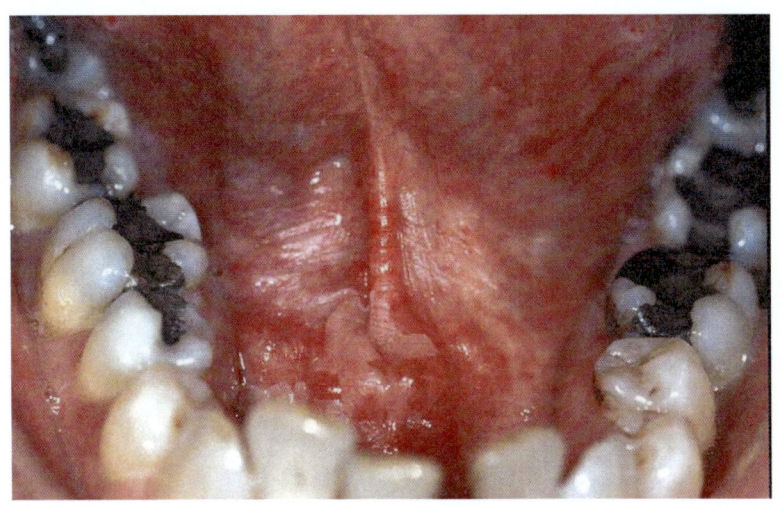

Fig. 100.3.

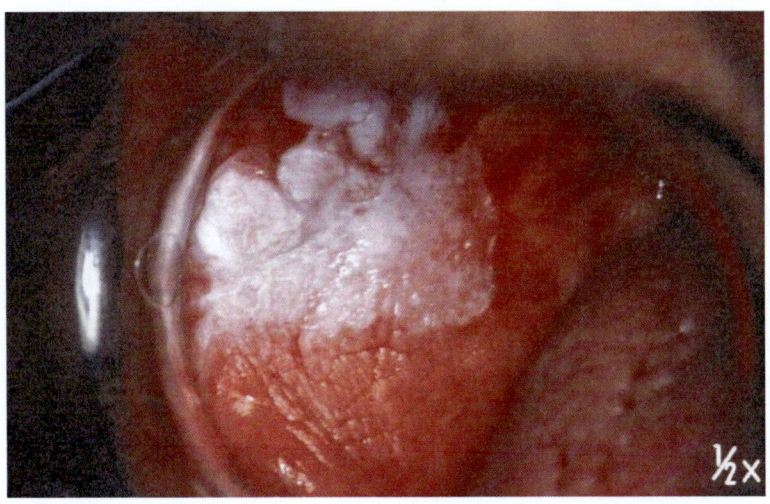

Fig. 100.4.

101. Lichen ruber planus oralis

Definition: Lichen ruber planus is a chronic inflammatory disease of the skin and mucous membranes.

Aetiology: Unknown

Symptoms: Stinging and burning. This occurs especially in the red/atrophic types. The condition is chronic.

Clinical features: There are two types: 1) whitish, keratinized and 2) red, atrophic/erosive types. The first group is the most frequent. It typically occurs in the so-called reticular form with fine white striae arranged in a reticulated pattern, patchy with swirling strokes, Fig.101.1. In the second group that is atrophy and oedemas of the epithelium. Clinically there are an atrophic type, an ulcerous type and a bullous type. The changes are mostly in the cheeks, tongue, Fig.101.2, palate and gingiva, Fig.101.3. The gingiva shows a desquamative gingivitis, which is very inconvenient for the patient, as it compromises the cleaning of the teeth.

Diagnosis: Performed clinically and by biopsi.

Treatment: Requires treatment only if there are symptoms. The condition is often infected with candida. Treatment starts with the antifungal treatment. After two weeks, the local steroid therapy is started, which for 2 weeks runs parallel to the fungal treatment. After completion of the antifungal treatment, the steroid treatment is continued for another 2 weeks. After the symptoms disappear, this is wound down.

Differential diagnosis: Leukoplakia. Discoid lupus erythematosus. Benign mucosal pemphigoid.

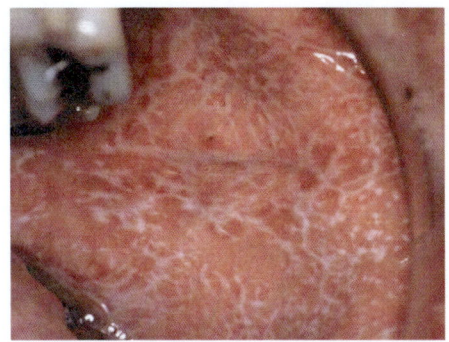

Fig. 101.1.

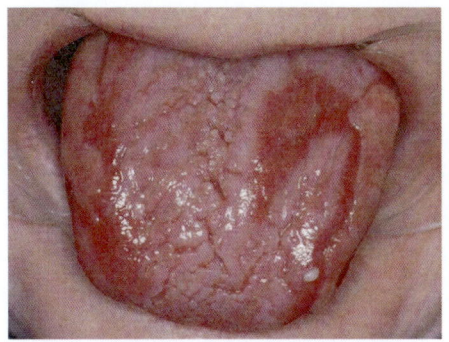

Fig. 101.2.

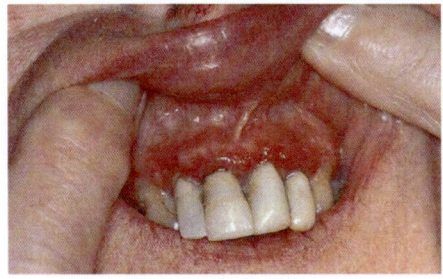

Fig. 101.3.

213

102. Lingua crenata (lingua indentata)

Also called Lingua indentata. Condition where teeth impressions are seen in the lateral edge of the tongue. Mostly due to a bad habit or macroglossia, as a result of acromegaly or amyloidosis. Fig.102.1.

103. Lingua fissurata

The furrowed tongue is also known as lingua scrotalis, lingua dissekta, lingua plicata or simply grooved tongue. The cause is unknown, but it is often associated with Down's syndrome and Melkersson- Rosenthal syndrome. Fig.103.1 and Fig.103.2.

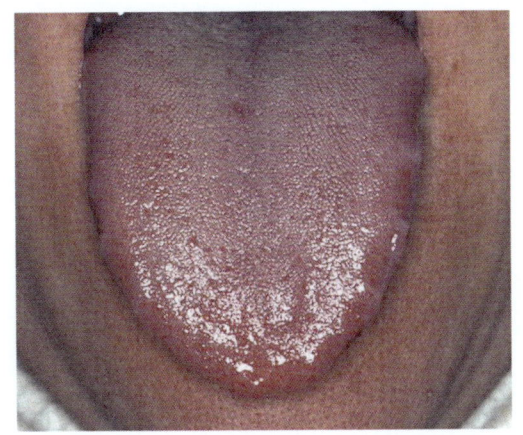

Fig. 102.1.

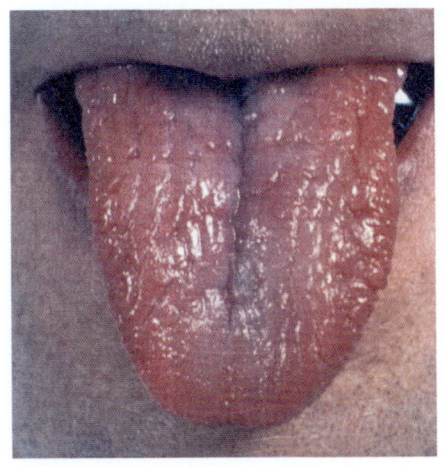

Fig. 103.1.

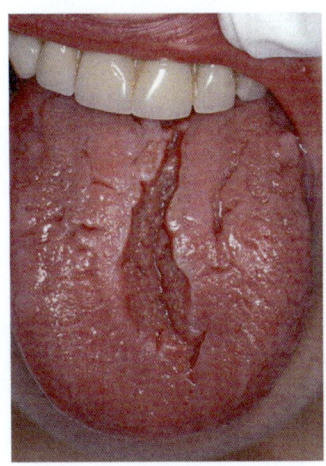

Fig. 103.2.

215

104. Lingua geografica

Definition: A benign condition with erythema migrans due to papilla loss in one or more areas on the dorsum of the tongue or margo.

Aetiology: Unknown. Ca. 4% is associated with psoriasis.

Symptoms: Often asymptomatic, but some cases involve discomfort with acidic and spicy foods.

Clinical features: There is a smooth erythema, bounded by raised, yellow-white markings, which often has a scalloped configuration. These red areas are due to papillary atrophy and seem to wander around on the surface of the tongue, Fig.104.1 and Fig.104.2.

Diagnosis: Performed clinically.

Treatment: Requires no treatment. In the event of symptoms and discomfort, try to relieve the superficial inflammation with mouthwashes and topical treatment with steroid cream.

The patient should be informed of the benign nature of the condition.

Differential diagnosis: Candidiasis.

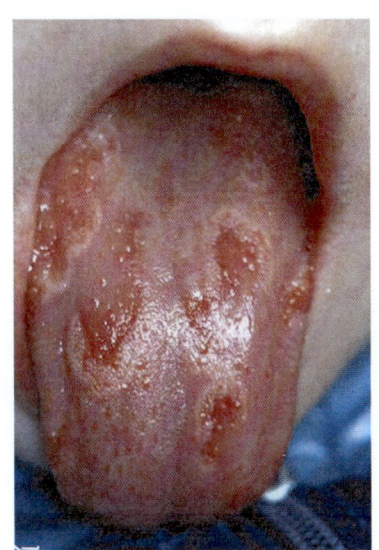

Fig. 104.1.

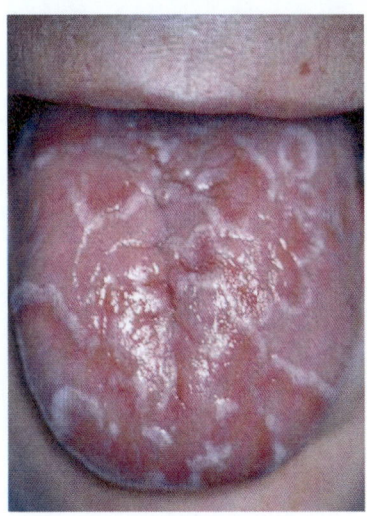

Fig. 104.2.

105. Lipoma

Definition: Benign tumour of the fat cells.

Aetiology: Unknown.

Symptoms: None. Slowly growing swelling.

Clinical features: Yellowish swelling with a smooth surface. When it is deep-lying, it feels hard, since it has a capsule. The most frequent tumour in the body, but rare in the oral cavity. In the mouth it is frequently seen in the cheek and in the tongue. Fig.105.1, Fig.105.2 and Fig.105.3.

Diagnosis: Histology

Treatment: As a rule it is easy to remove surgically because it has a capsule. Recurrence is rare.

Differential diagnosis: Fibroma. Myxoma. Mucocele. Neuro-fibroma. Leiomyoma.

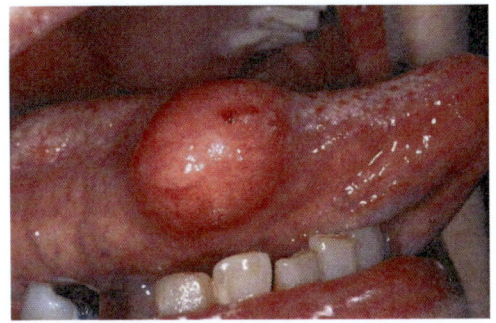

Fig. 105.1.

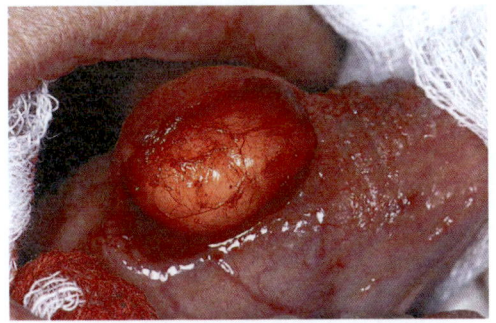

Fig. 105.2.

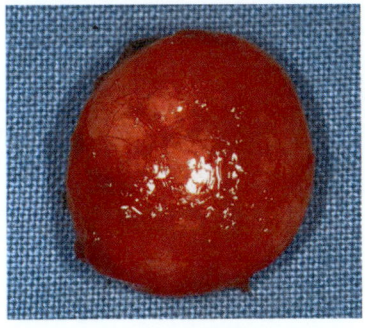

Fig. 105.3.

106. Lupus erythematosus, discoid

Definition: Chronic immunological skin and mucous membrane disorder.

Aetiology: Autoimmune.

Symptoms: Painful spicy foods, delicate mucous membranes which easily tear.

Clinical features: Lupus can occur in a systemic form (SLE) and a discoid form (DLE) with about 20-25% of patients having intraoral symptoms almost always accompanied by skin changes. The so-called discoid lesions are in typical cases characterised by a central atrophic reddish area with a slightly elevated, keratinized boundary, in which there are white thin irradiating striae (feather marking). In the red central area white, keratinized spots and possibly teleangiectasias can be seen. Seen most commonly on the cheeks, gingiva and prolabium. Fig.106.1 and Fig.106.2.

Diagnosis: Biopsy of intraoral lesion.

Treatment: Diagnosis and treatment carried out in collaboration with a dermatologist. The treatment is generally steroid therapy. The intra-oral lesions may be treated with additional local steroid cream.

Differential diagnosis: Lichen ruber planus. Lingua geografica. Benign mucous membrane pemfigoid. Erythroplacia. Candidiasis.

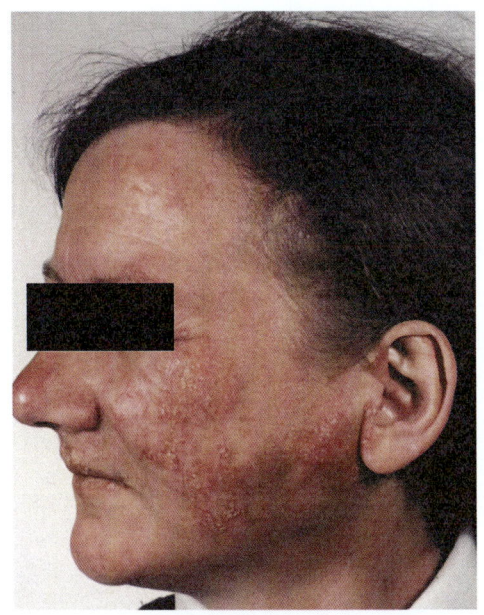

Fig. 106.1.

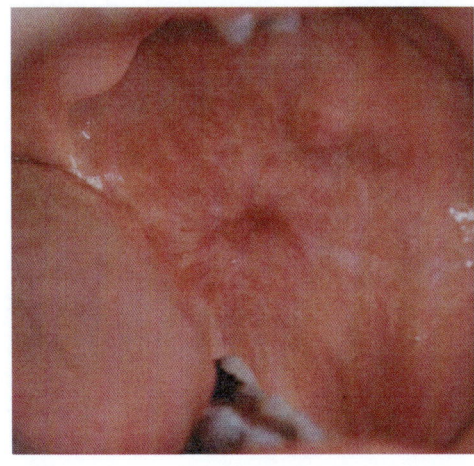

Fig. 106.2.

107. Lymphangioma

Definition: Benign hamartomatous tumour formed by the lymphatic vessels.

Aetiology: Unknown. It is debatable whether it is a real neoplasm or a developmental defect.

Symptoms: Eating and swallowing problems.

Clinical features: Most cases are thought to be innate or developed early after birth. Most frequent in children and adolescents. In the mouth it is most frequently seen on the front 2/3 of the tongue. Grows slowly toward puberty and can be undisturbed for many years. Usually superficially located, similar to the accumulation of frog eggs, small vesicles, which may be blood-filled and therefore can be confused with a hemangioma. A deeper tumour can present as a soft, poorly defined mass. Most frequent in men. Fig.107.1, Fig.107.2 and Fig.107.3.

Diagnosis: Performed on the clinical profile and medical history. Cannot be "blanched" with a glass slide, thereby distinguished from a hemangioma.

Treatment: Surgical removal with subsequent histology. Recurrence is frequent. The lymphangioma does not respond to sclerosing substances, as the hemangioma does.

Differential diagnosis: Hemangioma. Papilloma. Myoblastoma. Rhabdomyoma. Neurilemmoma.

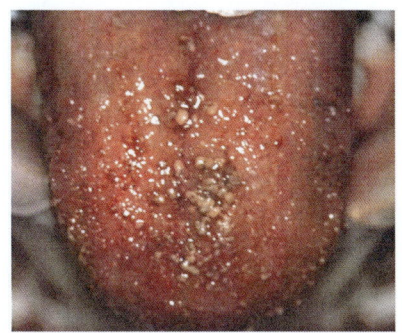

Fig. 107.1.

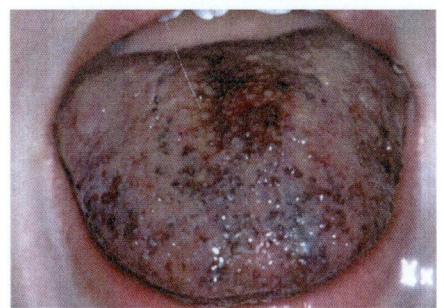

Fig. 107.2.

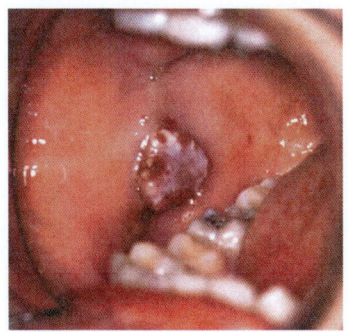

Fig. 107.3.

108. Lymphoma malignant (non-Hodgkin's lymphoma)

Definition: Malignant disease developed in the extranodal tissue.

Aetiology: Unknown

Symptoms: Swelling of the cervical lymph nodes. Intraorally swelling is seen in the hard palate and gingiva. Rapid growth, soft, meaty tissue prone to ulceration.

Clinical features: Fast-growing swelling, bleeding, ulceration. Tooth loosening. Under X rays large osteolytic processes are seen. Fig.108.1, Fig.108.2.

Diagnosis: Biopsy of an intra-oral lesion will often lead to the diagnosis.

Treatment: Refer to an oncology department. The treatment will be chemotherapy and/or radiation therapy.

Differential diagnosis: Mb. Hodgkins. Adenoidcystic carcinoma. Necrotizing sialometaplasia. Squamous cell carcinoma.

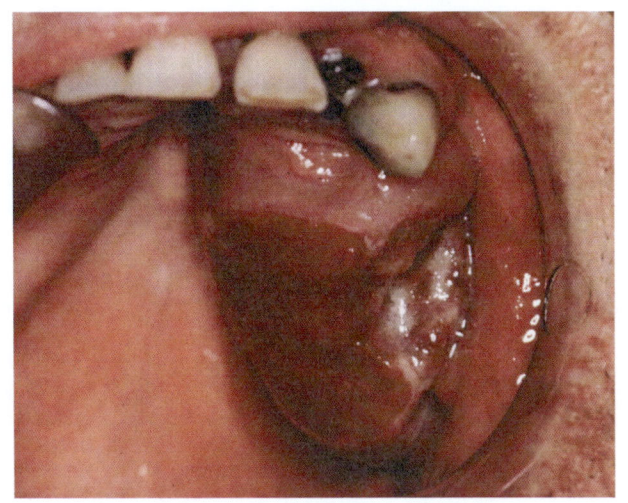

Fig. 108.1.

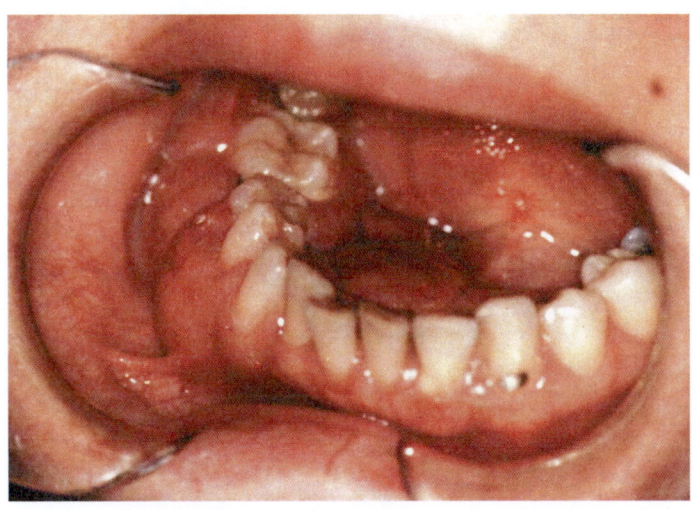

Fig. 108.2.

225

109. Melkersson-Rosenthal syndrome

Definition: Syndrome composed of: Paralysis of facial nerve, swelling of the upper lip and lingua plicata.

Aetiology: Unknown.

Symptoms: When mature it involves hanging mouth angle and lack of facial expression. Swelling of the upper lip and heavily fissured tongue.

Clinical features: Affects men and women with equal frequency. Seen most commonly in spring and autumn. In the oral cavity gingival swelling can be seen, in particular, corresponding to the interdental papillae. The syndrome can be seen in incomplete form. Fig.109.1, Fig.109.2.

Diagnosis: Performed on a lip biopsy.

Treatment: The bulky lips can be treated with steroid injections.

Differential diagnosis: Other granulomatous disorders Angio-oedema.

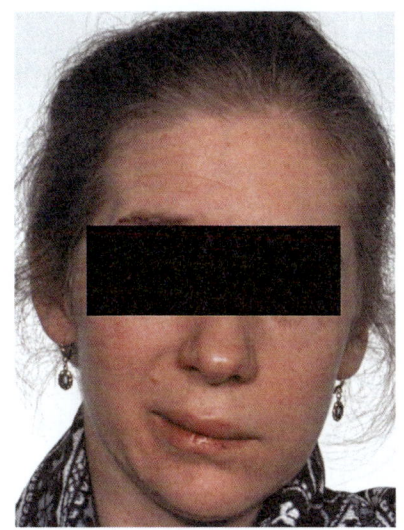

Fig. 109.1.

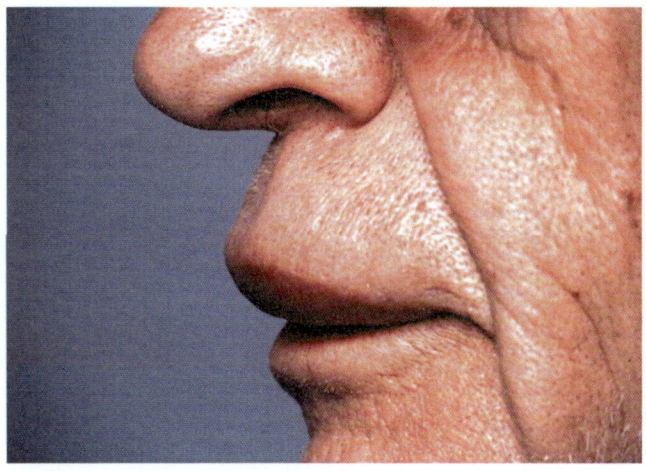

Fig. 109.2.

110. Morbus Osler

Definition: Hemorrhagic teleangiectasias.

Aetiology: Congenital defect.

Symptoms: Cosmetic irritation, frequent bleeding. Fatigue and weakness due to gastrointestinal bleeding. Seen frequently in the transition between the skin and mucous membrane.

Clinical features: Perioral lesions, pink, violet or purple in colour. It is seen in the tongue, palate, gingiva and buccal mucous membrane. Frequent nosebleeds. There is a defect in the capillaries and small blood vessels, characterised by dilation of the small blood vessels, which are free of elastic tissue. Fig.110.1, Fig.110.2. Not to be confused with phlebectasia linguae as seen in Fig.110.3.

Diagnosis: Performed on the clinical profile, medical history and histological examination.

Treatment: Refer to the dermatologist. Intraorally troublesome bleeding can be stopped with cryosurgery or laser therapy.

Differential diagnosis: Phlebectasia linquae (sublinqual varices). Chronic liver disease.

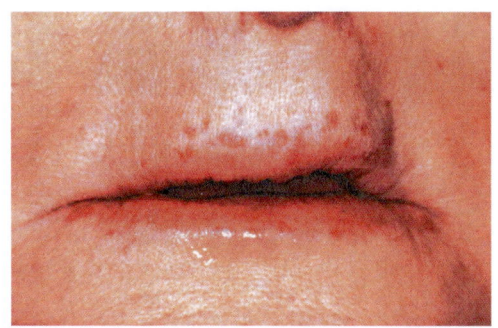

Fig. 110.1.

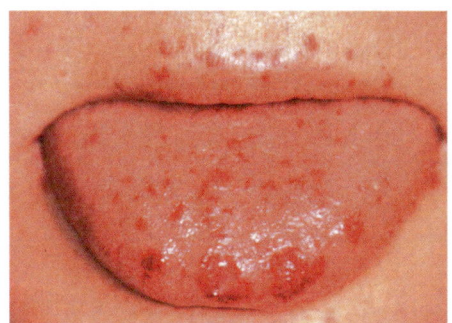

Fig. 110.2.

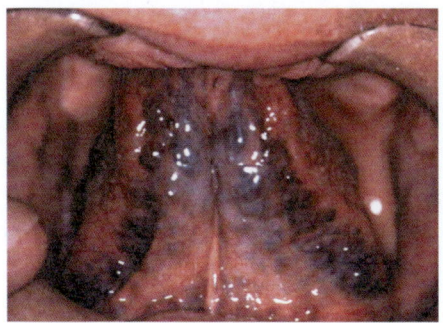

Fig. 110.3.

111. Morsicatio buccarum

Definition: Ulceration along the bite plane in the cheek.

Aetiology: Bad habit of chewing on the buccal mucous membrane. Stress effects.

Symptoms: Pain and bleeding, possibly with infections.

Clinical features: Parafunctions are well known in the dental field. The mucous membrane is rough and frayed. Cheek biting, tongue biting, lip biting and bruxism are all parafunctions. Often there are quite large destructions with infection in the area. Stings and burns from the consumption of spicy foods. Fig.111.1, Fig.111.2 and Fig.111.3.

Diagnosis: Performed by medical history and clinical examination.

Treatment: Discontinue the habit. Instruction in tongue exercises possibly with an acrylic shield on a bite splint for the protection of the cheek.

Differential diagnosis: Leukoplakia. Candidiasis. Hairy Leukoplakia. Carcinoma.

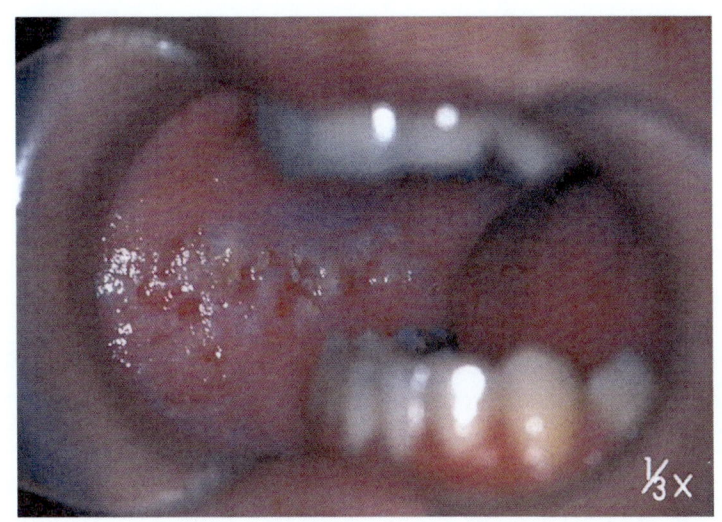

Fig. 111.1.

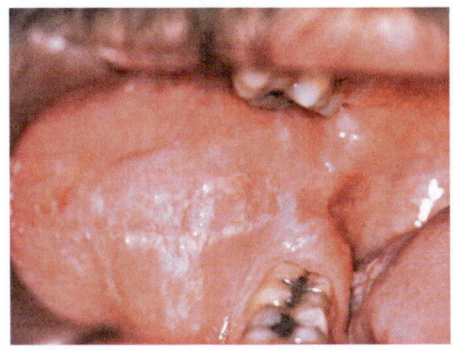

Fig. 111.2.

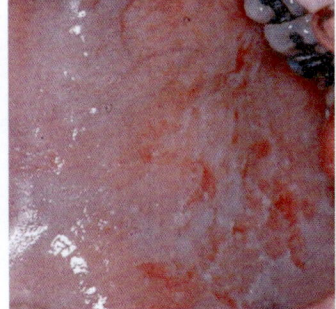

Fig. 111.3.

231

112. Mouth cancer (Cancer in the oral cavity)

Definition: Cancer of the oral cavity.

Aetiology: Suspicions of tobacco and alcohol. The cancer risk is dose-and time-dependent. Alcohol and tobacco appear to have a synergistic effect.

Symptoms: There may be soreness, pain and irritation from the tumour. In advanced tongue cancer there may be impaired mobility of the tongue and referred pain in the neck or ears. In addition, there may be paresthesia. In a few cases, swollen lymph nodes in the neck will be the symptom that causes the patient to be examined.

Clinical features: The mucous membrane can be seen with red sores with hardened circles and a smooth or nodular surface. For more advanced tumours, it is possible to see an exophytic process with a red/white, nodular and sometimes ulcerated surface. Fig.112.1, Fig.112.2. Sometimes there is a large ulcer with a central necrosis. With tongue cancer, the tongue can become fixed. The primary locations are the tongue side edges, floor of the mouth and alveolar process in the lower jaw, Fig.112.3.

Diagnosis: The diagnosis is performed on a biopsy.

Treatment: Referral must be made to a larger centre. Surgery and/or radiation therapy are the treatments.

Differential diagnosis: Saliva gland tumour. Lymphoma. Kaposi's sarcoma. Metastasis.

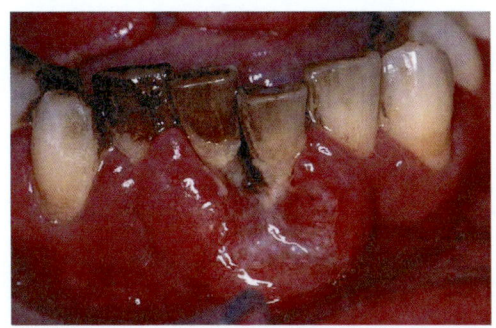

Fig. 112.1.

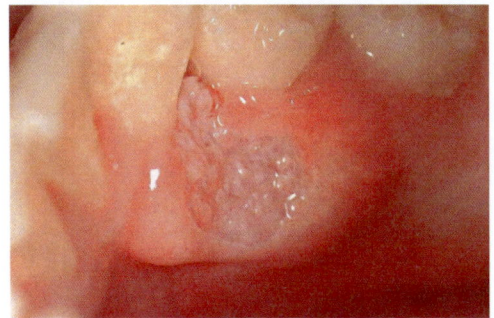

Fig. 112.2.

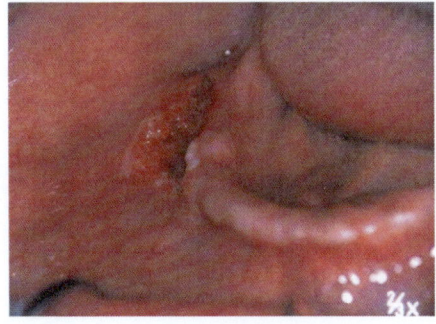

Fig. 112.3.

Lip cancer - cancer labii:

The most frequent oral cancer in the Western world. Seen most commonly in older men.

Clinical features: Ulceration, swelling. Most commonly in the lower lip. Very varied appearance. Fig.112.4, Fig.112.5. Fig.112.6. shows a cancer occurring in an **actinic elastosis**.

There is induration on palpation of the tumour.

Diagnosis: The clinical profile and biopsy.

Treatment: Referral to specialised department. Surgical removal. The prognosis is good.

Differential diagnosis: Keratoacanthoma. Actinic elastosis.

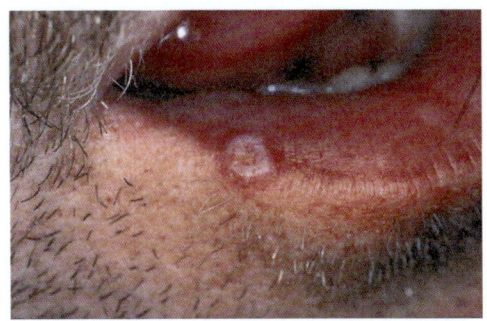

Fig. 112.4.

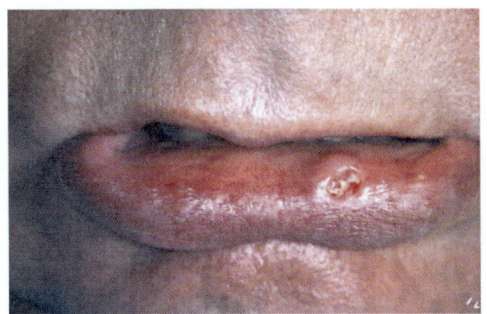

Fig. 112.5.

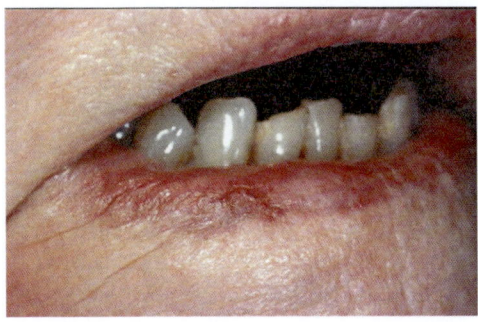

Fig. 112.6.

Metastases:

Metastases to the mouth and jaw occur relatively infrequently. Only about 1% of malignancies in the oral region are metastases from other organs. The organs in which metastases to the mouth are frequently seen are, in declining order of frequency: the breasts, lungs, kidney, gl.thyreoidea, prostate, colon, gastric, testis, bladder, cervix uteri and ovaries. In the oral region metastasis to the jaws is the most frequent. In a major study it was found that soft tissue metastase represents approximately 14% of all metastases to the oral region. The most frequent location is the gingiva where half of the soft tissue metastases are found.

Fig.112.7 shows a metastasis from a breast carcinoma.

Fig.112.8 shows a metastasis from a lung cancer.

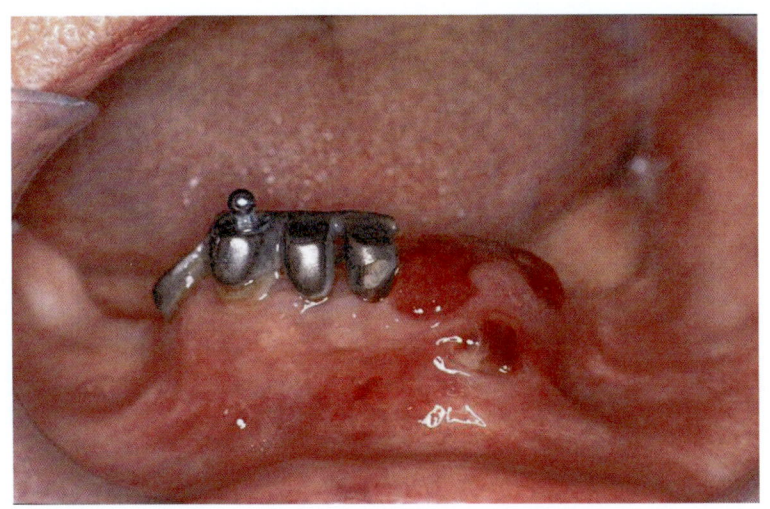

Fig. 112.7.

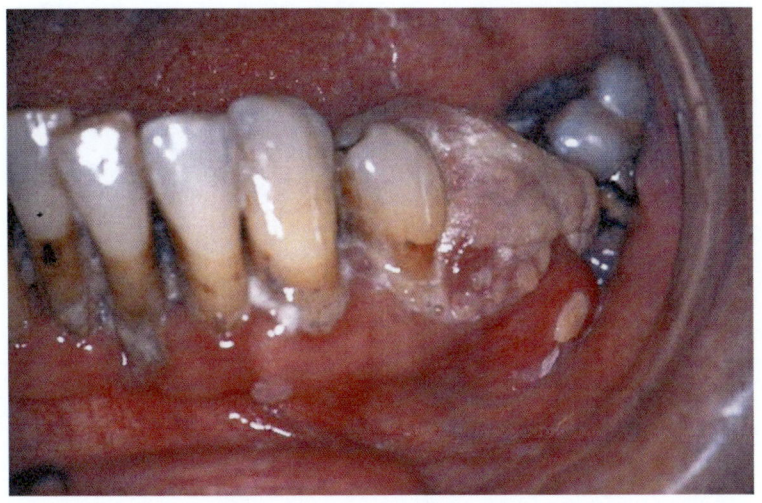

Fig. 112.8.

113. Multiple myeloma

Definition: Rare malignant plasma cell disease.

Aetiology: Unknown.

Symptoms: Expansion of the bone, dental loosening, pain and paresthesia.

Clinical features: Most common in men over 50 years. The jaws are involved in 30% of cases. There can be painless soft swelling on proc.alveolaris and gingiva. Fig.113.1 and Fig.113.2

Diagnosis: Biopsy, blood, bone marrow biopsy.

Treatment: Chemotherapy, radiation therapy.

Differential diagnosis: Plasmacytoma. Non-Hodgkin's lymphoma. Ewing's sarcoma.

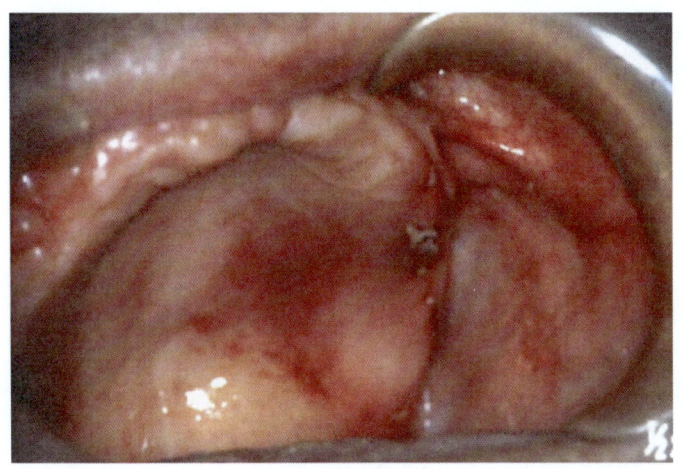

Fig. 113.1.

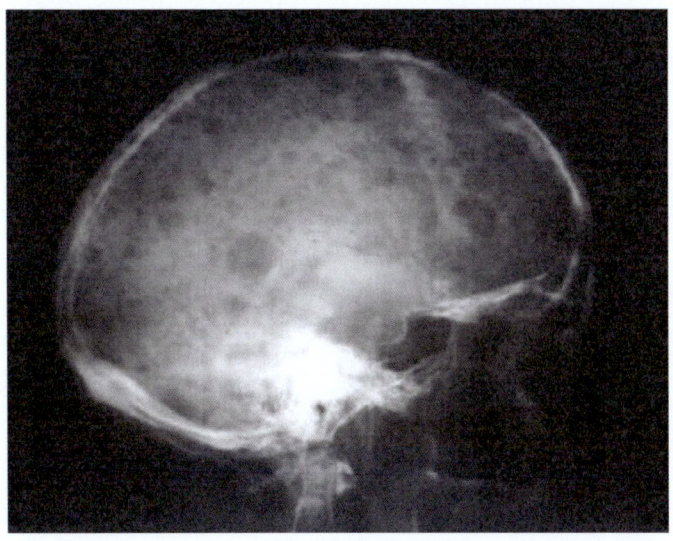

Fig. 113.2.

114. Myoblastoma granulare

Definition: Benign soft tissue tumour. It is debatable whether it is a neoplasm.

Aetiology: Unknown.

Symptoms: Swelling of the tongue. Rarely pain.

Clinical features: Most often seen in the oral cavity and there most frequently in the tongue. Appears as a solid, submucosal nodule on the dorsum. Varies considerably in size. The mucous membrane can be pink to yellowish, with normal surface, rarely ulcerated. Fig.114.1.

Diagnosis: Performed by a biopsy.

Treatment: Surgical removal.

Differential diagnosis: Fibroma. Lipoma.

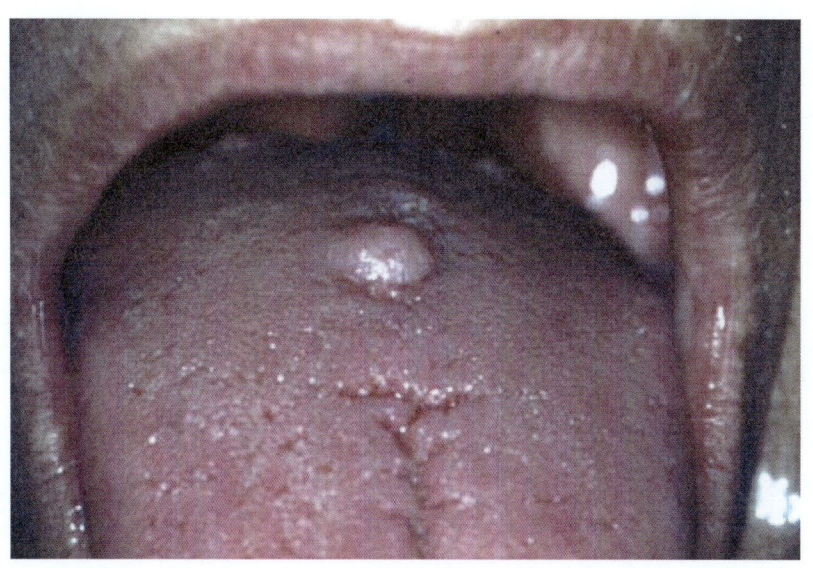

Fig. 114.1.

115. Myxoma odontogenica

Definition: Benign tumour arising in odontogenic mesenchymal tissue.

Aetiology: Unknown

Symptoms: No or asymptomatic swelling.

Clinical features: Most frequently in younger people, 25-30 years. Evenly divided between the sexes. Most frequently seen in the mandible. Often discovered during a routine x-ray. Fig.115.1 and Fig.115.2.

Diagnosis: Performed on the radiological image and biopsy.

Treatment: Curettage, but larger lesions require resection, since the disorder is locally aggressive. Does not metastasize .

Differential diagnosis: Cysts. Neurofibroma.

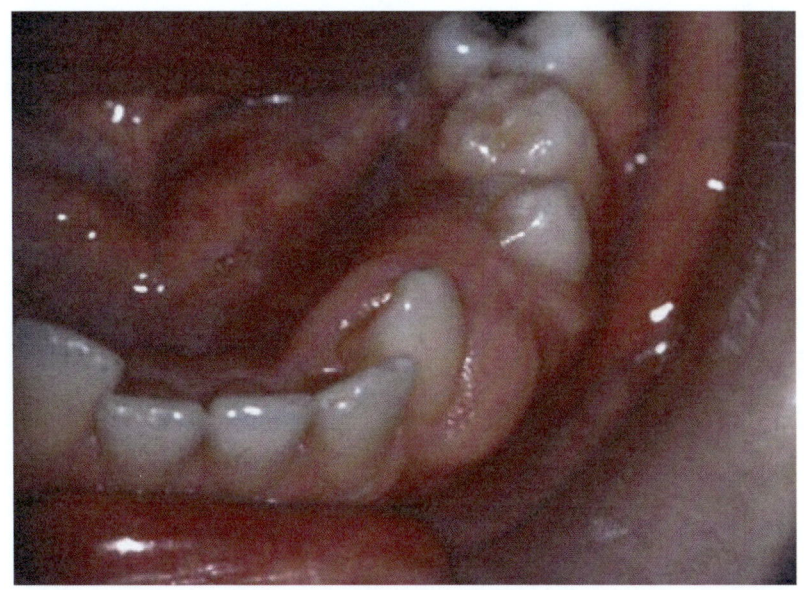

Fig. 115.1.

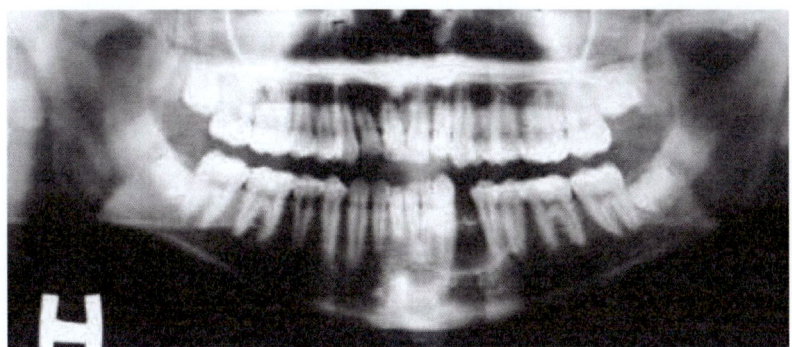

Fig. 115.2.

116. Naevus albus spongiosus: (White sponge naevus)

Definition: Rare, inherited disorder. Benign. Termed genodermatosis.

Aetiology: Unknown, inherited autosomal dominant.

Symptoms: Symmetrical, white coatings with a spongy appearance.

Clinical features: Appearing at birth or in early childhood. Occurs in families. Buccal mucous membrane and tongue are most frequently affected. Fig.116.1, Fig.116.2 and Fig.116.3.

Diagnosis: Clinical and biopsy.

Treatment: None

Differential diagnosis: Leukoedema. Leukoplakia. Lichen planus. Cheek biting.

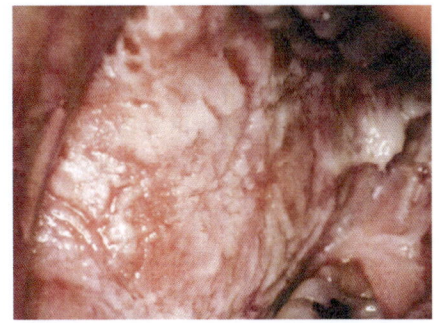

Fig. 116.1.

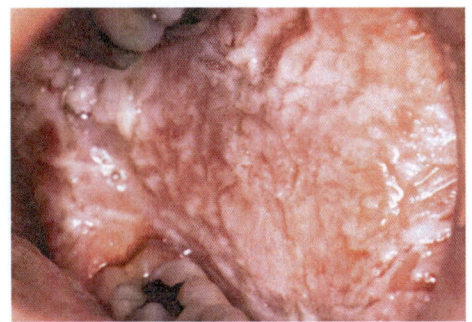

Fig. 116.2.

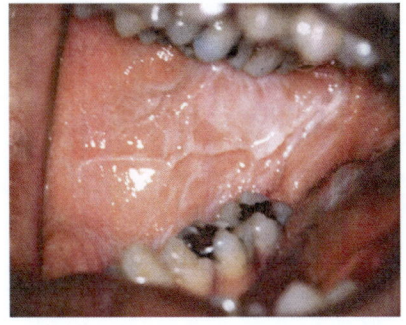

Fig. 116.3.

117. Neurofibromatosis

Definition: Benign neoplasm originating from the Schwann cells or perineural cells.

Aetiology: Unknown.

Symptoms: Swelling of the skin or mucous membrane. No pain.

Clinical features: Well-defined, solid, broad-based or pedunculate swelling. Covered with normal epithelium. The size varies from 0.5 to 1.5 cm. Most frequent in the tongue, cheek and palate. Fig.117.1, Fig.117.2 and Fig.117.3. Multiple neurofibromas are seen with **Neurofibromatosis von Recklinghausen**.

Diagnosis: Performed after biopsy.

Treatment: Surgical removal. Neurofibromatosis von Recklinghausen requires referral to specialist care

Differential diagnosis: Fibroma. Schwannoma. Granular cell tumour.

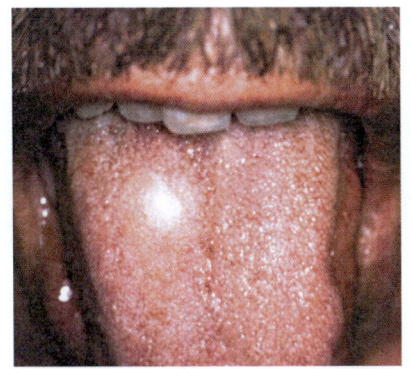

Fig. 117.1.

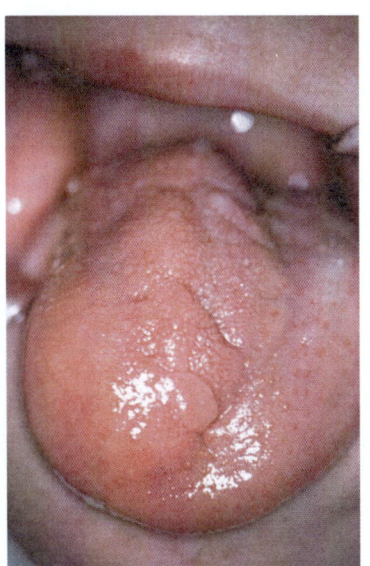

Fig. 117.2.

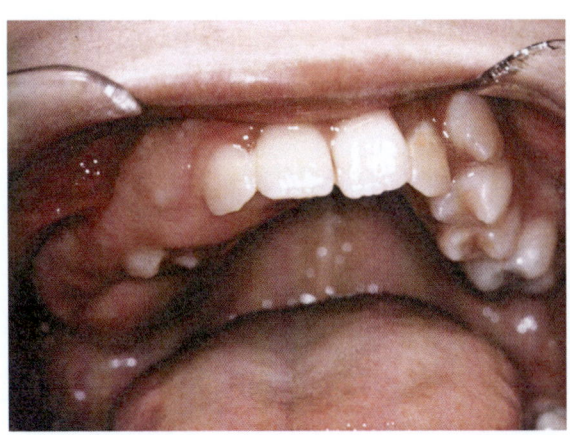

Fig. 117.3.

118. Neutropenia cyclica

Definition: Rare hematological disorder characterised by cyclic reduction in the number of neutrophil granulocytes.

Aetiology: Congenital or unknown! The most serious type called agranulocytosis develops on an immunological basis or through a causative agent.

Symptoms: Malaise, neck pain, fever. Headache, joint pain and pain from the gastrointestinal tract.

Clinical features: Orally there are painful punched wounds covered by white fibrin membranes. Fig.118.1, Fig.118.2 and Fig.118.3.

Diagnosis: Refer to GP. Performed by blood test.

Treatment: Any triggering factor discontinued. Antibacterial treatment.

Differential diagnosis: Aphtae. Granulocytosis. Leukaemia. Aplastic anaemia.

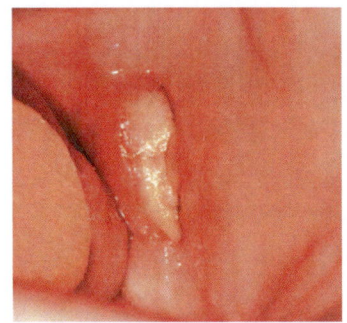

Fig. 118.1.

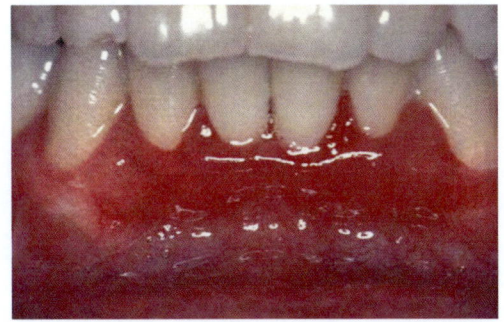

Fig. 118.2.

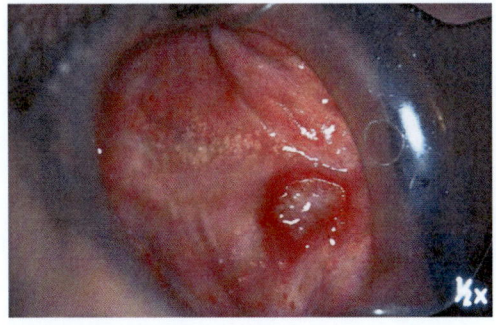

Fig. 118.3.

119. Ossifying fibroma

Definition: Reactive gingiva proliferation with a distinctive histo-pathological appearance. Also called fibroblastic granuloma with ossification and ossifying fibrous epulis and peripheral fibroma with ossification.

Aetiology: Unknown, but is thought to develop from the parodontal ligament or periosteum.

Symptoms: None. Bleeding from the gingiva.

Clinical features: Exclusively on the gingiva. Most commonly in children, adolescents and women. A well-defined solid swelling, broad-based or stalked. Often covered by normal mucous membrane. Most commonly in the front and canine region. The size varies from 0.5 to 2 cm. Fig.119.1, Fig.119.2 and Fig.119.3.

Diagnosis: Performed on histological examination.

Treatment: Surgical removal.

Differential diagnosis: Fibroma. Pyogent granuloma. Giant cell granuloma. Granuloma gravidarum.

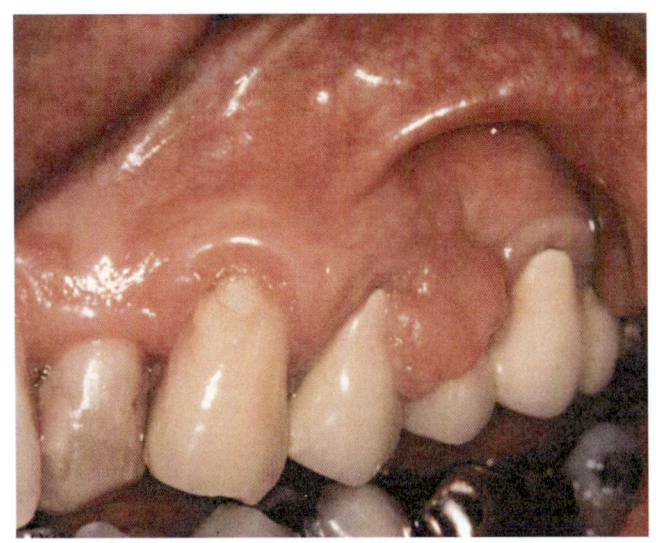

Fig. 119.1.

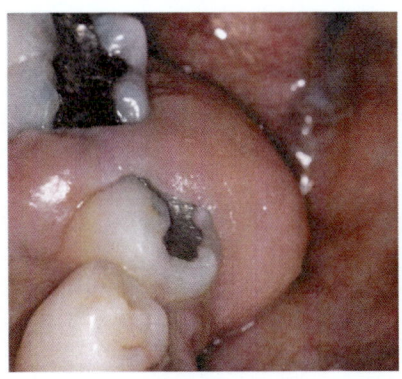

Fig. 119.2.

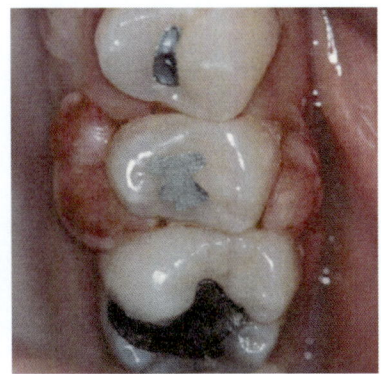

Fig. 119.3.

120. Osteoma

Definition: Benign tumour composed of mature cortical or spongy bone.

Aetiology: Unknown.

Symptoms: Slow-growing swelling. No pain.

Clinical features: The swelling of the bone may vary in size from a few millimetres to several centimetres. Fig.120.1 and Fig.120.2.

Diagnosis: Performed on radiological suspicion and histological examination.

Treatment: Surgical removal.

Differential diagnosis: Exostoses. Osteosarcoma.

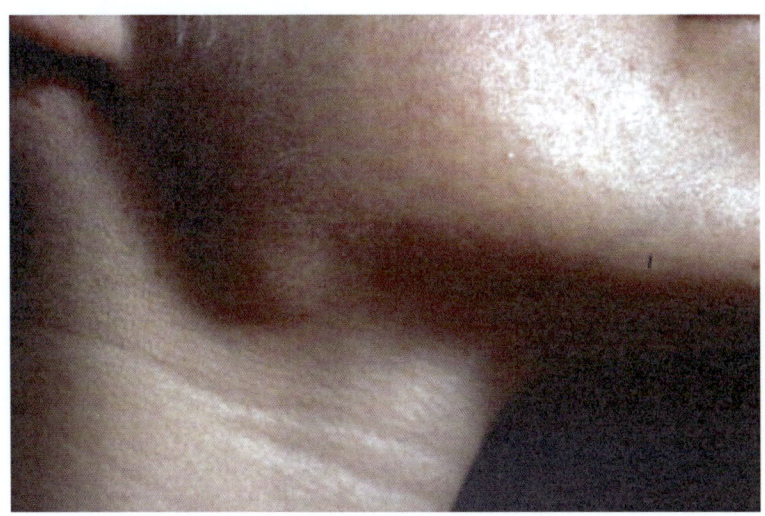

Fig. 120.1.

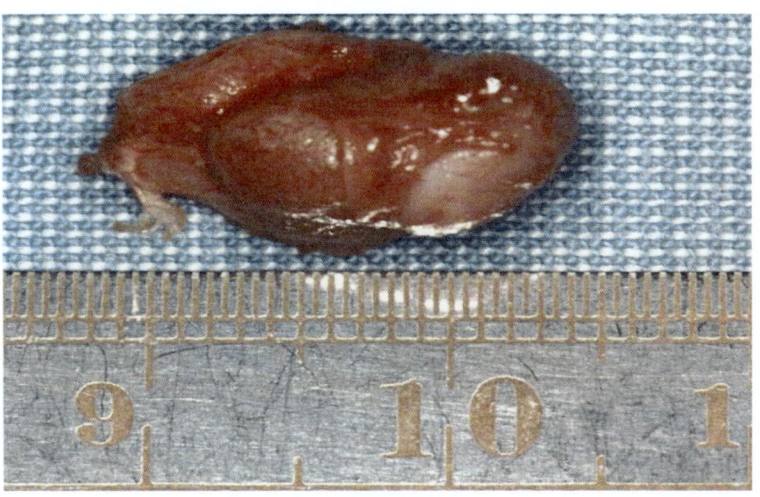

Fig. 120.2.

121. Osteomyelitis

Definition: Chronic inflammation of the jawbone.

Aetiology: Bacterial penetration. Most frequently periodontitis, fracture sequelae or sequelae after radiotherapy. Termed osteo-radionecrosis.

Symptoms: Pus, pain, formation of sequestra.

Clinical features: Slow-growing expansion of the bone. In the acute stage painful. There may be malaise. Fig.121.1 and Fig.121.2

Diagnosis: Performed on the radiological image, clinical examination and possibly a swap.

Treatment: Prolonged antibiotic treatment is often targeted at anaerobic microorganisms possibly with combined substance therapy.

Differential diagnosis: Osteoradionecrosis. Chemotherapy sequelae. Other general disease with decreased resistance as a result.

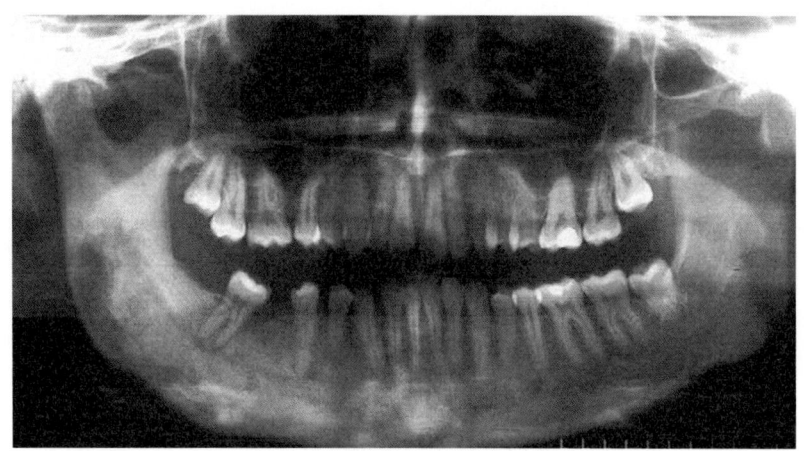

Fig. 121.1.

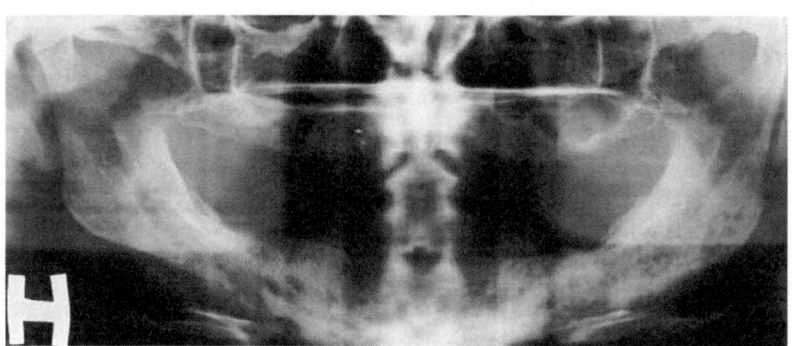

Fig. 121.2.

122. Papilloma

Definition: Benign tumour originating from the squamous epithelium.

Aetiology: Unknown.

Symptoms: None.

Clinical features: Occurs in all age groups. Most frequently in women. Most common on the tongue, buccal mucous membrane and gingiva. True neoplasm, which is often stalked, with small finger-like proliferations, which give it a cauliflower-like appearance. Usually well-defined, but may be considerable. Slowly growing. Degenerate very rarely malignant. Fig.122.1, Fig.122.2 and Fig.122.3 Clinical tumour cannot be distinguished from the virus-induced Verruca Vulgaris.

Diagnosis: Performed clinically and histologically after removal.

Treatment: Surgical removal.

Differential diagnosis: Verruca vulgaris. Condyloma acuminatum.

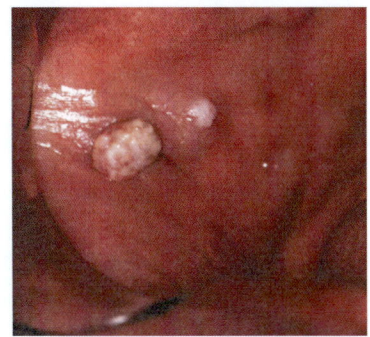

Fig. 122.1.

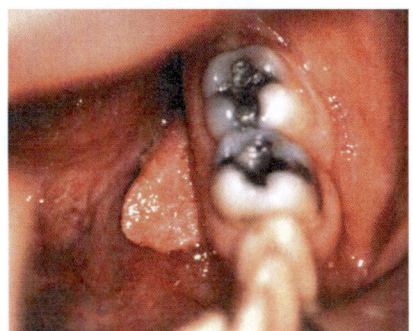

Fig. 122.2.

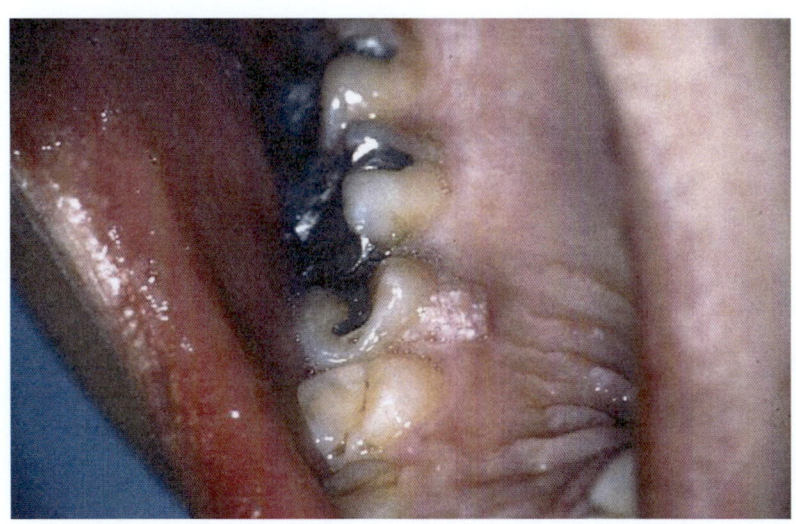

Fig. 122.3.

123. Pemphigus

Definition: Chronic bullous autoimmune mucocutaneous disease.

Aetiology: Autoimmune disorder. Autoantibodies directed against the desmosomes in the epithelium, leading to intraepithelial bullae formation.

Symptoms: There are 4-6 types, of which P.vulgaris is the most frequent. The skin exhibits limp bullae, which can appear anywhere. In the mouth there are also bullae and erosions that predominate. Pain.

Clinical features: 70% of cases start in the mouth. Painful blisters which rapidly burst. Most commonly in the 40-60 years age range, equal frequency in men and women. Characteristic is **Nikolsky's sign**, which means that the bulla can be squeezed out of the normal mucous membrane. Fig.123.1, Fig.123.2 and Fig.123.3.

Diagnosis: Performed on the basis of the clinical signs, histology and immune fluorescence study of normal tissue.

Treatment: Refer to the Department of Dermatology. Steroid. Untreated, the disease can be fatal.

Differential diagnosis: Pemphigoid. Erythema multiforme. Bullous lichen.

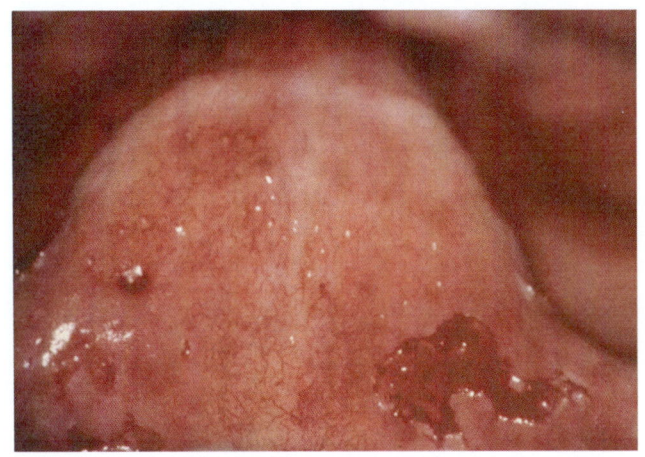

Fig. 123.1.

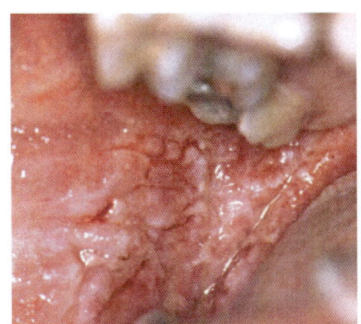

Fig. 123.2.

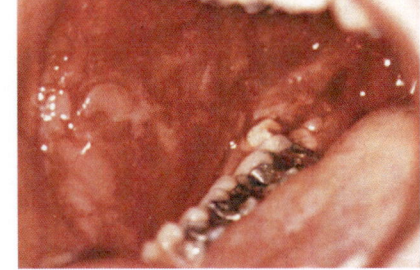

Fig. 123.3.

124. Perimylolysis

Definition: Acid damage of the palatal side of the teeth.

Aetiology: Acid reflux, regurgitation, rumination.

Symptoms: Sensitive teeth, loss of tooth substance, loss of interocclusal distance.

Clinical features: Acid-washed teeth, rounded shapes on the molars. Very sensitive to cold. Fig.124.1. Acid damage can also be seen with excess citric intake Fig.124.2 and with excess Cola drinking, also Fig.124.3.

Diagnosis: Performed from the medical history and the clinical profile.

Treatment: Crown treatment for the conservation of the interocclusal distance. Preventive treatments. Perhaps suspected bulimia, anorexia. Reference to the doctor for investigation.

Differential diagnosis: None.

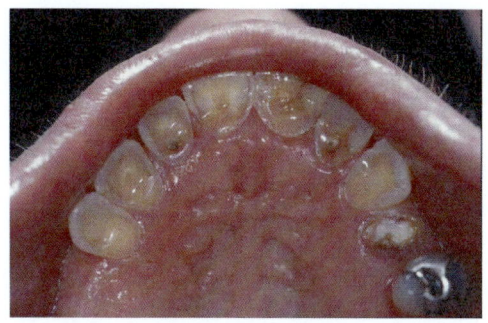

Fig. 124.1.

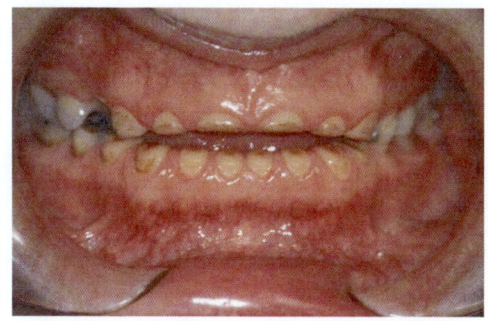

Fig. 124.2.

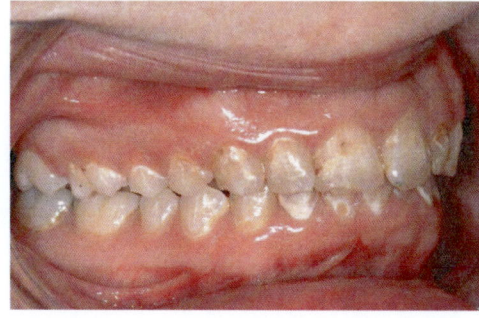

Fig. 124.3.

125. Periodontitis (periodontal disease)

Definition: A chronic infectious disease of the teeth suspensory apparatus.

Aetiology: Poor hygiene. A combination of several bacterial strains (in particular a number of gram-negative and anaerobic strains).

Symptoms: Patients will experience bleeding and flow of pus from the gums and possibly abscess formation. The teeth will be long and possibly wander. There will often be bad breath because of high plaque volumes and dental calculus.

Clinical features: Plaque and dental calculus. Bad breath, Fig.125.1 and Fig.125.2. Bleeding and flow of pus from the pocket. The teeth will be long and loose and have changed position. An X-ray will reveal loss of the alveolar bone. In a very small group of young patients (< 1%), the disease progresses particularly rapidly. This condition is termed aggressive periodontitis or juvenile periodontitis. It is likely that patients with periodontitis marginalis are at increased risk of developing cardiovascular disease.

Diagnosis: Performed clinically and on X-rays.

Treatment: Treatment and frequent monitoring. Dental root cleaning, as well as training and close monitoring of the patient's oral hygiene. Possibly additional surgery.

Differential diagnosis: Hematological disease.

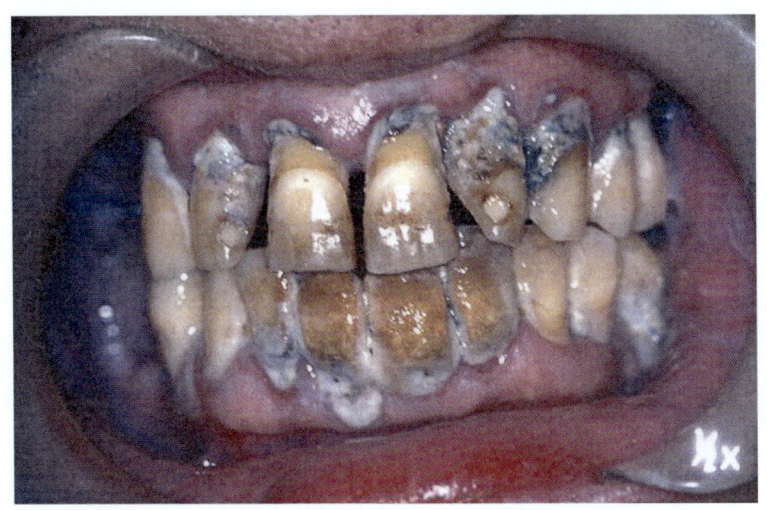

Fig. 125.1.

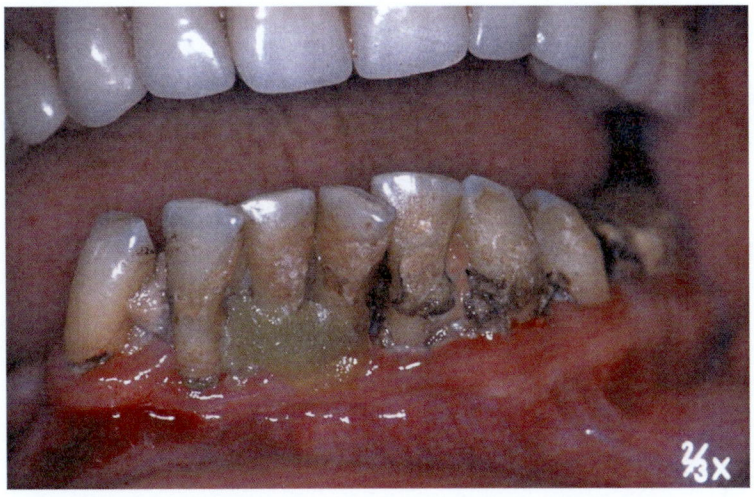

Fig. 125.2.

263

126. Quincke's oedema

Definition: The Quincke's oedema is a diffuse, oedematous swelling of the soft tissues.

Aetiology: Probably a degranulation of the mast cells with subsequent histamine release.

Symptoms: Difficulty in breathing because of swelling of the tongue, which is soft and without pain. Perioral and periorbital swelling is typical.

Clinical features: Hypersensitivity reaction may also occur as a contact allergic reaction or due to physical stimuli. Visible oedematous elements in the face. Fig.126.1, Fig.126.2 and Fig.126.3.

Diagnosis: Performed on the clinical profile and medical history.

Treatment: Antihistamines. Refer to GP. In acute cases ensure free airways.

Differential diagnosis: Melkersson-Rosenthal syndrome. Mb.Crohn.

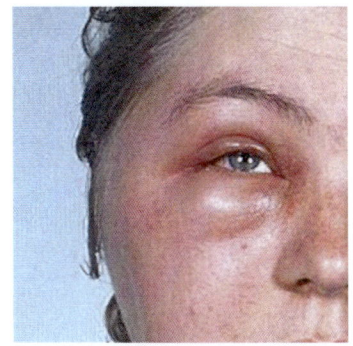

Fig. 126.1.

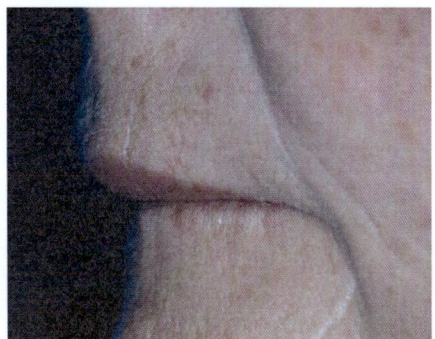

Fig. 126.2

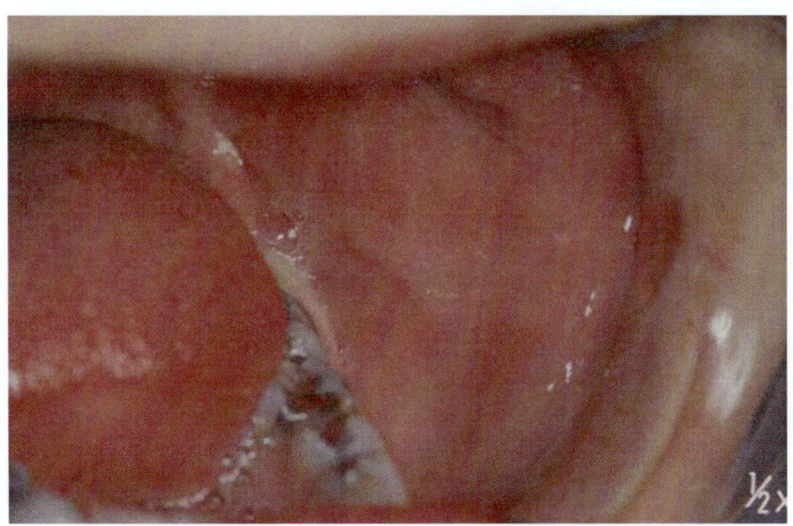

Fig. 126.3.

127. Ranula

Definition: Soft tissue cyst occurring exclusively in the floor of the mouth. The name comes from the similarity with the belly of a frog.

Aetiology: Obstruction of the duct or trauma.

Symptoms: Swelling before meals. Mild pains.

Clinical features: Fluctuating swelling, depending on the saliva production. Moderate pain. Fig.127.1, Fig.127.2 and Fig.127.3.

Diagnosis: Performed on the clinical profile and medical history and biopsy of the removed tissue.

Treatment: Extirpation or marsupialisation.

Differential diagnosis: Dermoid cyst. Lymphangioma.

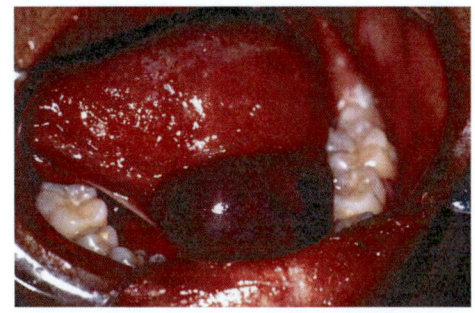

Fig. 127.1.

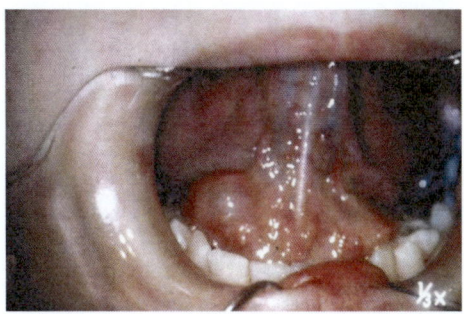

Fig. 127.2.

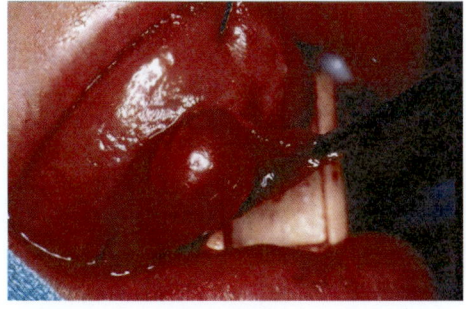

Fig. 127.3.

128. Sarcoidosis

Definition: Multisystemic, granulomatous disease.

Aetiology: Unknown.

Symptoms: Difficulty breathing. Dry cough. Chest pain, fever, fatigue. Joint pains and weight loss.

Clinical features: Intraorally there are uncharacteristic swellings. In rare cases bone involvement. Fig.128.1 and Fig.128.2

Diagnosis: Performed on histological examination.

Treatment: Refer to the dermatologist. High doses of steroids.

Differential diagnosis: Crohn's disease. Heerfordt's syndrome.

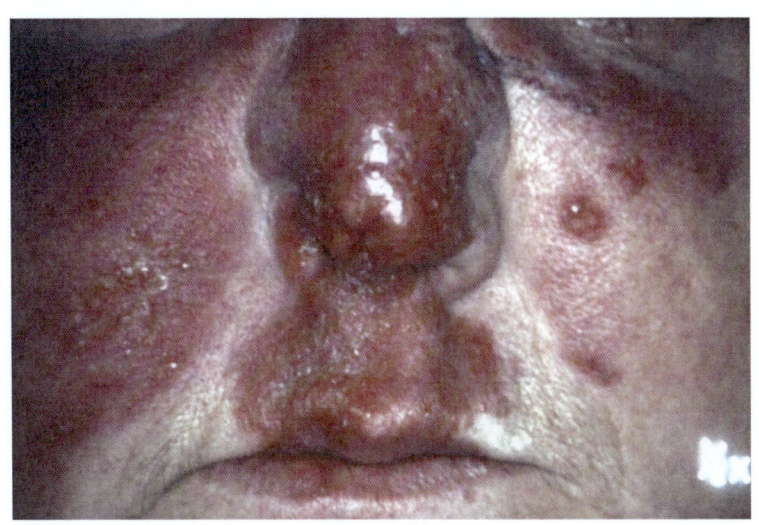

Fig. 128.1.

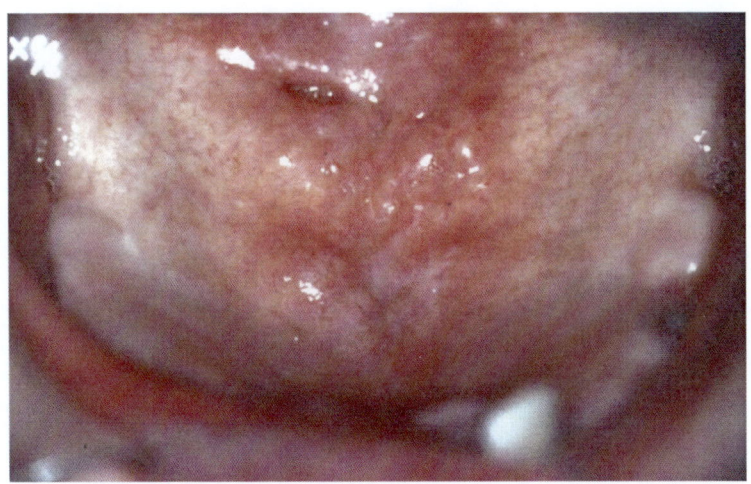

Fig. 128.2.

129. Scleroderma

Definition: Progressive, chronic sclerosis of the connective tissue with an immunological features.

Aetiology: Unknown.

Symptoms: Thickening and induration of the skin. Teleangiectasias. Arthralgia. Myopathies. Nephropathy.

Clinical features: Periorally tighter and tighter skin is observed around the mouth, with strong narrowing of the rima oris. Radiating furrows around the mouth. Pronounced trace of the parodontal cleft around the teeth. Dental treatment almost impossible. Fig.129.1 and Fig.129.2.

Diagnosis: Referral to a specialist unit. Blood Test. X-ray.

Treatment: Penicillin. Steroids. Possibly anti-hypertension treatment.

Differential diagnosis: Mixed connective tissue disease. Rheumatoid Arthritis.

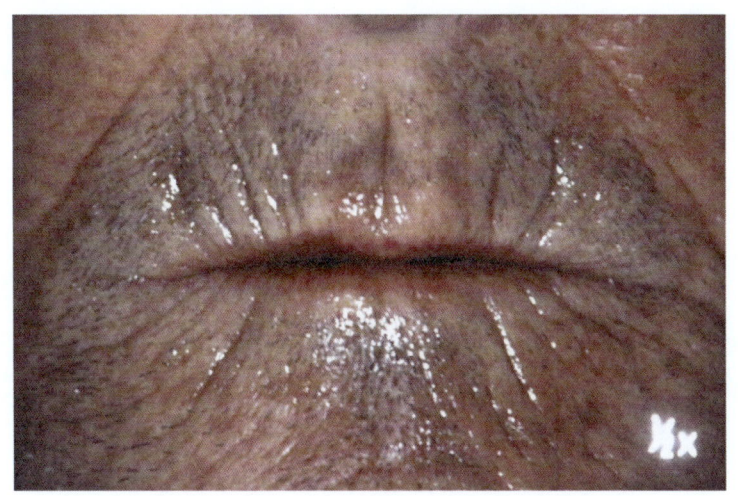

Fig. 129.1.

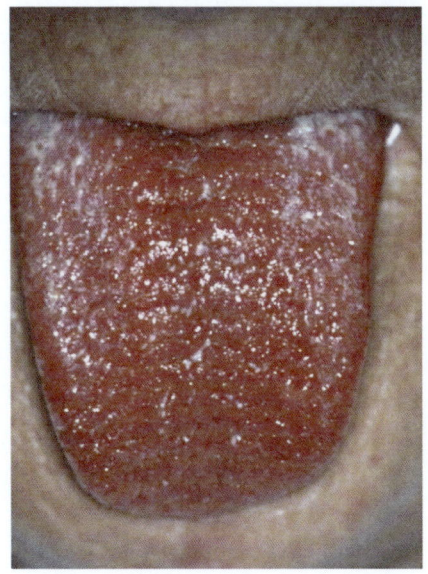

Fig. 129.2.

271

130. Sequestrum

Definition: A piece of avital bone.

Aetiology: Either sequelae of operation or pathological disorder.

Symptoms: None.

Clinical features: The bone becomes exfoliated after about three months. Bad smell and taste. Bad breath. Fig.130.1 and Fig.130.2.

Diagnosis: Performed clinically.

Treatment: Surgical debridement of the dead tissue.

Differential diagnosis: Serious general diseases. Osteomyelitis.

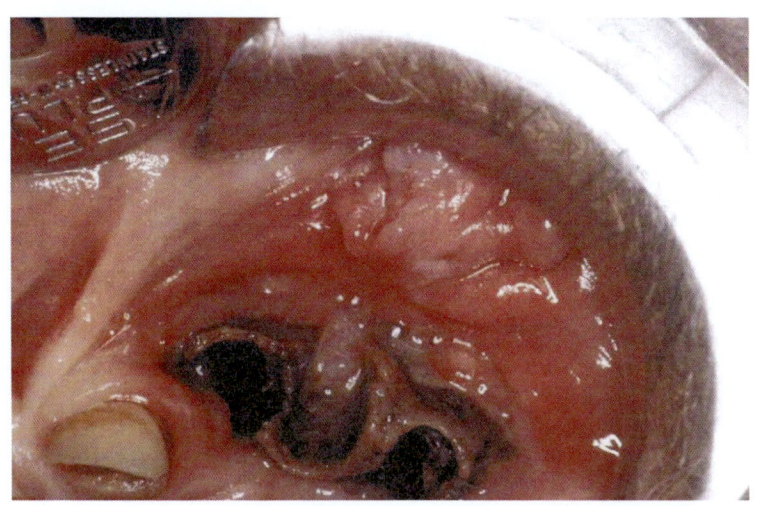

Fig. 130.1.

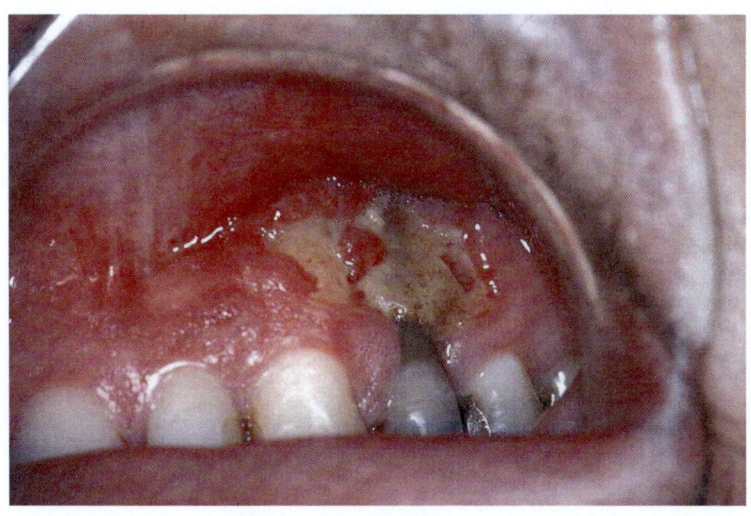

Fig. 130.2.

131. Sialolithiasis

Definition: Calcifications in the ductus of the gland or in the gland resulting in infection.

Aetiology: Salivary stone (sialolith). When saliva is accumulated in the duct there is inflammation with a risk of infection.

Symptoms: Swollen lymph nodes, sialoadenitis, pus in the duct and swollen gland.

Clinical features: Swelling, often meal-related, malaise, often visible salivary stones. Most commonly in relation to gl. sub-mandibularis. Fig.131.1, Fig.131.2 and Fig.131.3.

Diagnosis: Performed from the medical history and the clinical profile.

Treatment: Surgical removal of large stones. Small stones (e.g. in gl.parotis) can often be handled by dilatation of the duct with a silver probe.

Differential diagnosis: Saliva gland tumour. Sialoadenitis.

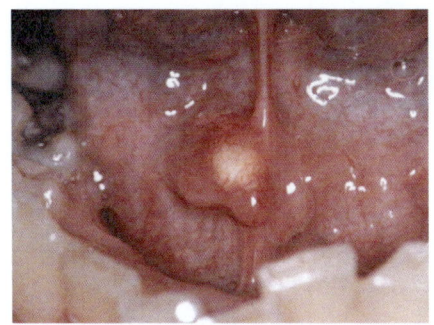

Fig. 131.1.

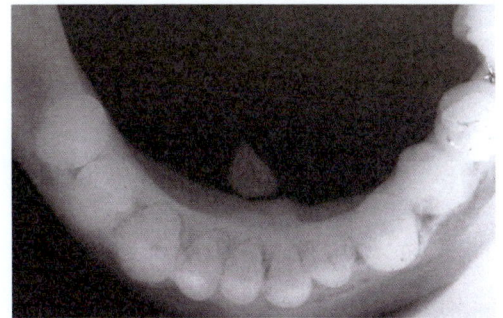

Fig. 131.2.

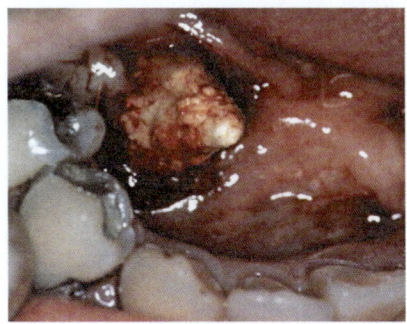

Fig. 131.3.

275

132. Smoker's palate (stomatitis nicotina palati)

Definition: Changes in the palate mucosa, caused by pipe smoking.

Aetiology: Pipe smoking

Symptoms: Normally none.

Clinical features: Clinically there is a palate mucous membrane, which is diffuse grey or white with numerous, slightly elevated excrescences in which a small red punctate area is centrally observed. These points represent the metaplastic changed ducts from the accessory salivary glands of the palate. The entire palatal keratinization can become so thick that the mucous membrane seems fissured, Fig.132.1.

Diagnosis: Performed clinically and by the medical history.

Treatment: None. The condition is not precancerous.

Differential diagnosis: Leukoplakia.

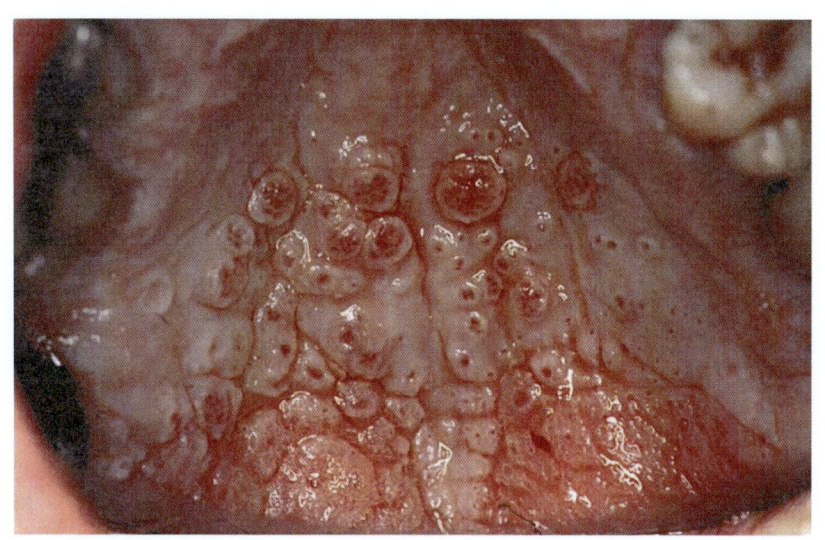

Fig. 132.1.

133. Steven-Johnson syndrome

Definition: Most serious form of Erythema multiforme exudativum.

Aetiology: Unknown.

Symptoms: Distressed general condition, fever, all mucous membranes affected. Dehydration. Arthralgia and myalgia.

Clinical features: Observed between 20-40 years age. Most frequently in men. In the mouth bullae are seen that rupture and lead to erosions. Fig.133.1. The eyes, Fig.133.2 and sex organs are also affected Fig.133.3. The condition lasts 2-6 weeks.

Diagnosis: Performed on the clinical profile and compounding of the symptoms.

Treatment: Local or systemic steroid therapy. Fluid therapy.

Differential diagnosis: Herpetic gingivostomatitis. Pemphigoid. Pemphigus. Erosive lichen planus.

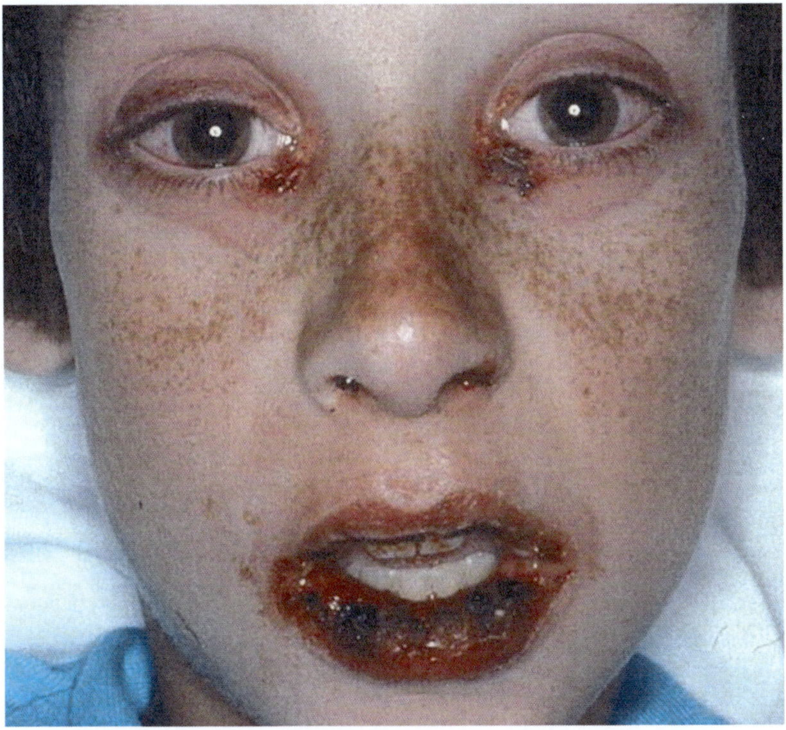

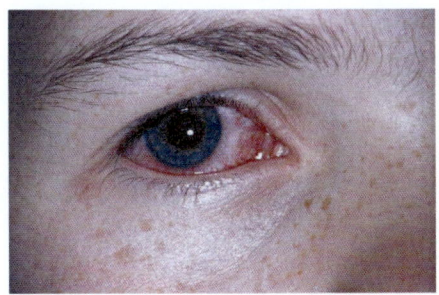

Fig. 133.1.

Fig. 133.2.

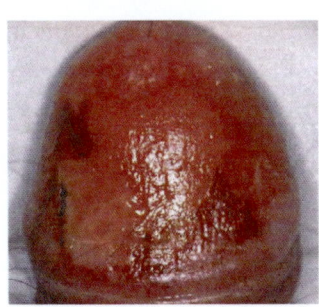

Fig. 133.3.

134. Stomatitis aphtosa recurrens cicatricicans

Definition: Deep wounds with a red halo surround, leaving scars.

Aetiology: Unknown, cell-mediated immune response.

Symptoms: The wounds can be 1-2 cm in diameter and last for 2-3 weeks before scarring. Very painful.

Clinical features: Patients are very pain-ridden when the wounds are fresh. There may be 1-5 at a time. The prevalence is 10-30%. Fig.134.1, Fig.134.2 and Fig.134.3.

Diagnosis: Performed from the medical history and the clinical profile.

Treatment: Local treatment for infection and pain. Possibly intralesional steroid injections.

Differential diagnosis: Carcinoma. Cyclic neutropenia. Syphilis.

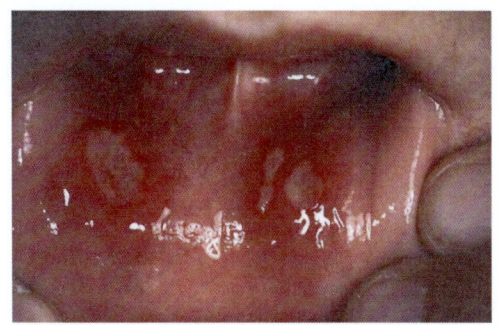

Fig. 134.1.

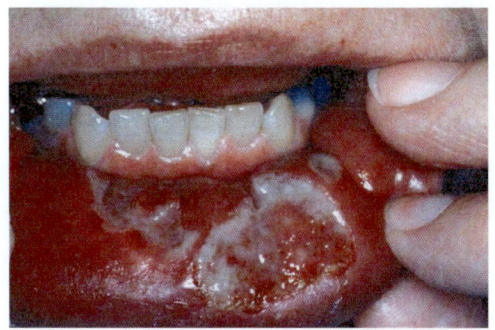

Fig. 134.2.

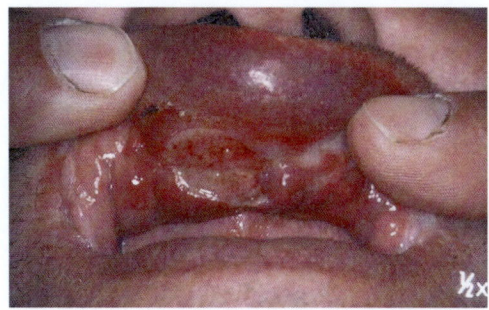

Fig. 134.3.

281

135. Stomatitis e radiatione

Definition: Reactive inflammation of the oral mucous membrane.

Aetiology: Therapeutic radiation treatment for head and neck.

Symptoms: Pain, fungal infection, ulceration, pain and burning, taste disturbance, difficulty swallowing, difficulty speaking. Dry mouth. Late complications of caries and osteoradionecrosis.

Clinical features: After a week of radiotherapy the mucous membrane appears greyish with oedema and hyper-keratinization. This is followed by erythema and after 3 weeks ulcerations are seen. The ulcerations confluence and the whole mucous membrane becomes a large wound. The radiation destroy the cells' normal "turn-over" and when the basal cells are most radiosensitive there is no renewal. Fig.135.1, Fig.135.2 and Fig.135.3.

Diagnosis: The medical history and the clinical profile allow the diagnosis.

Treatment: Specialist treatment in the acute phase. Camomile tea, chlorhexidine, antifungal treatment, local pain. Saliva stimulating agents (Xerodent). The discomfort will last for about 4-6 weeks after the end of treatment, but the dry mouth can often be lifelong.

Differential diagnosis: Erythema multiforme. Herpetic gingivo-stomatitis.

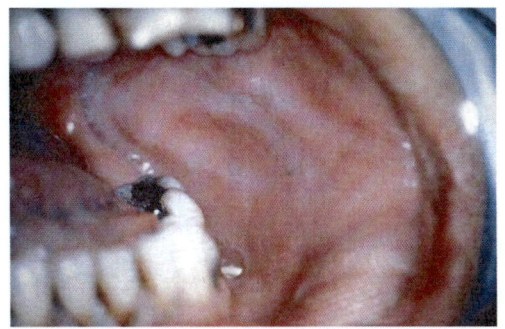

Fig. 135.1.

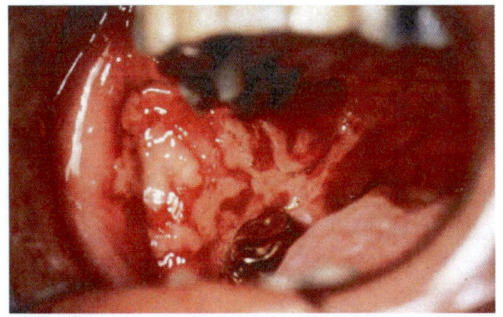

Fig. 135.2.

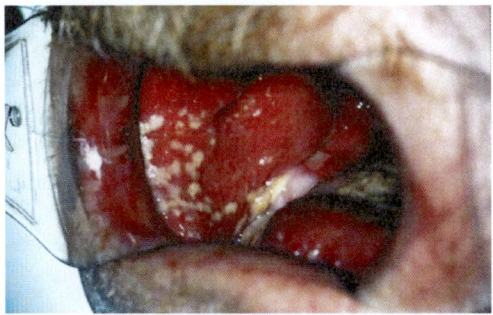

Fig. 135.3.

136. Thrombocytopenia

Definition: Haematological disorder characterised by a low platelet count in the peripheral blood.

Aetiology: Unknown. Perhaps a viral infection or a myelotoxic agent.

Symptoms: Bleeding from the mouth, nose, gastrointestinal tract and urinary tract.

Clinical features: Gingival bleeding is one of the earliest signs. Petechiae, suggilations, ecchymosis and haematomas can be seen. Fig.136.1, Fig.136.2 and Fig.136.3.

Diagnosis: Secured by blood sample, bleeding and clotting times.

Treatment: Steroids. Transfusion. Possibly removal of a causative agent.

Differential diagnosis: Aplastic anaemia. Leukaemia. Agranulocytosis. Polycythemia vera.

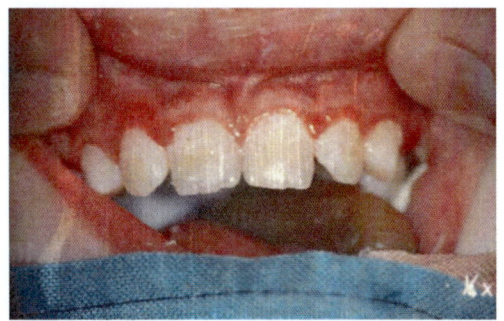

Fig. 136.1.

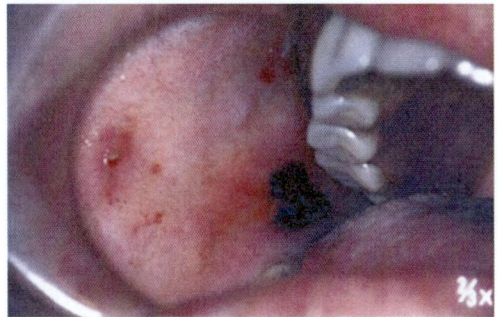

Fig. 136.2.

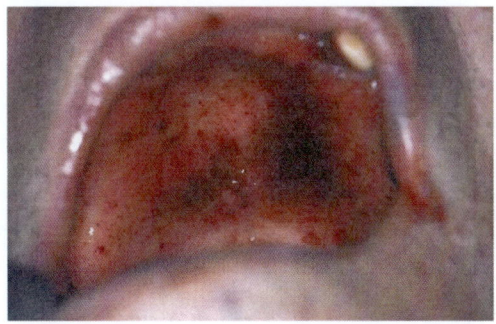

Fig. 136.3.

137. Torus mandibularis

Definition: Developmental malformation.

Aetiology: Unknown.

Symptoms: None. But may produce functional problems for denture carriers.

Clinical features: Asymptomatic bone swelling covered by normal mucous membrane. Bilateral of mandibular lingual side in the premolar region. But can also be facial. Fig.137.1, Fig.137.2.

Diagnosis: Performed clinically.

Treatment: None. With removable denture or discomforts, then surgical removal.

Differential diagnosis: Osteoma.

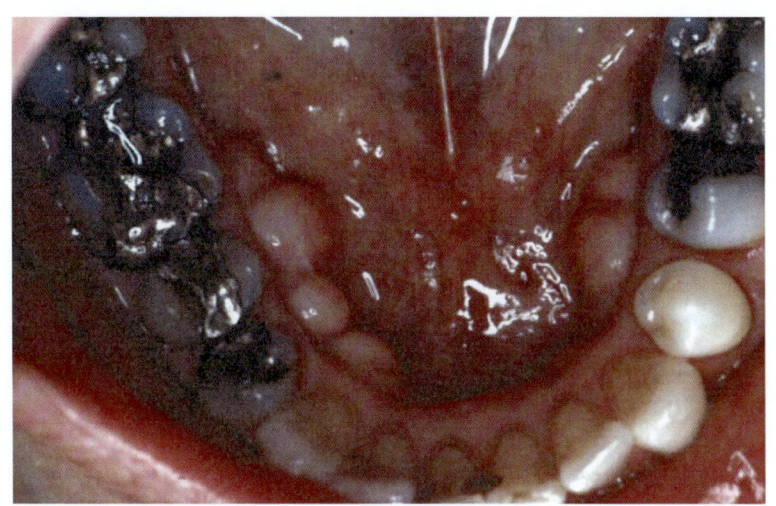

Fig. 137.1.

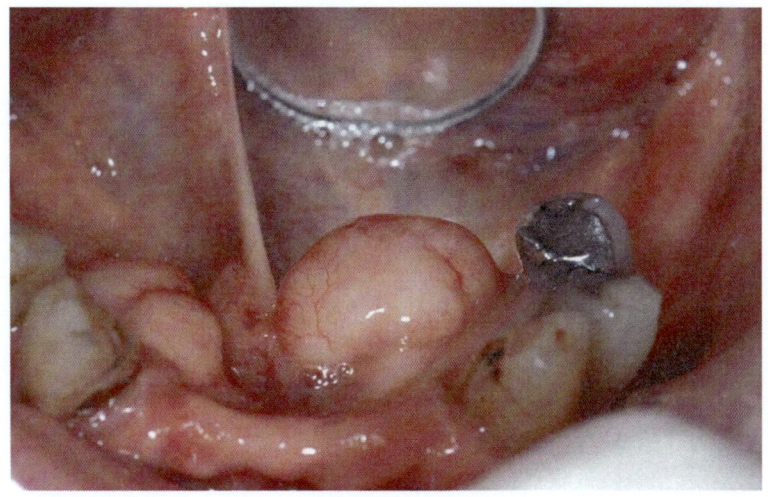

Fig. 137.2.

287

138. Torus palatinus

Definition: Developmental malformation.

Aetiology: Unknown.

Symptoms: None. With denture production it can cause functional problems.

Clinical features: Asymptomatic, slow-growing lobular or nodular swelling. Seen in the midline of the hard palate. Most frequent in women. Fig.138.1, Fig.138.2.

Diagnosis: Performed on the clinical profile.

Treatment: None. Possibly surgical removal in the event of discomforts.

Differential diagnosis: Osteoma.

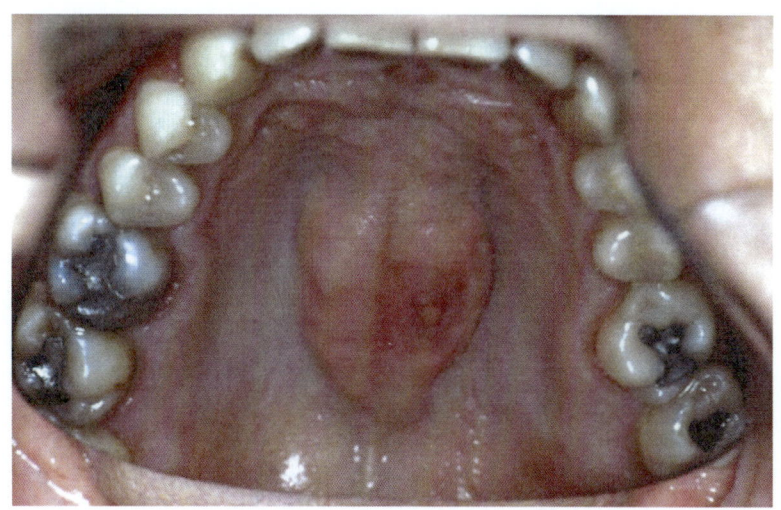

Fig. 138.1.

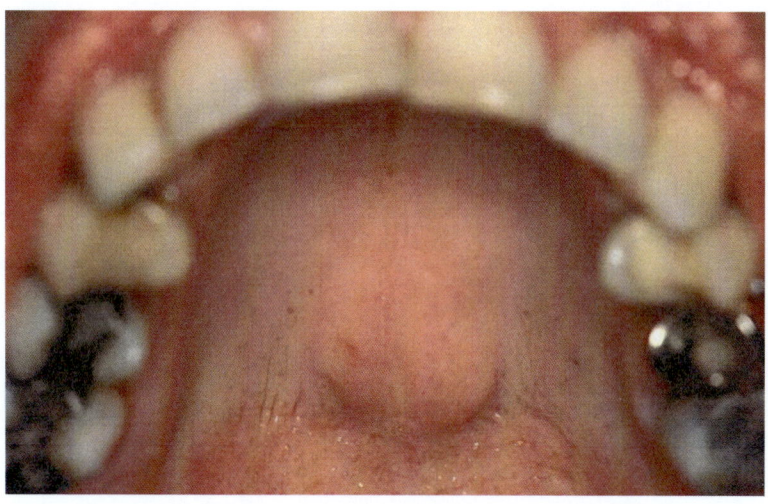

Fig. 138.2.

139. Tumor mucoepidermoides

Definition: Malignant tumour derived from salivary glands.

Aetiology: Unknown.

Symptoms: Asymptomatic to mild pain. Facial paresis. Swelling. Intraosseous radiolucency.

Clinical features: The most frequent malignant salivary gland tumour. Considered to be between 10-20% of salivary gland tumors. Occurs in all age groups. Most frequent in women. Most commonly in the palate, but also in the lip, tongue, floor of mouth and the retromolar area. The tumour may be ulcerated and may have a bluish tinge, so that it can be confused with a mucocele. Fig.139.1, Fig.139.2, Fig.139.3.

Diagnosis: Performed clinically and histologically after biopsy. Staging is performed in the light of the prognosis.

Treatment: Depending on the gradation of the tumour. Surgery, which includes resection in the event of bone involvement.

Differential diagnosis: Adenoidcystic carcinoma. Mucocele.

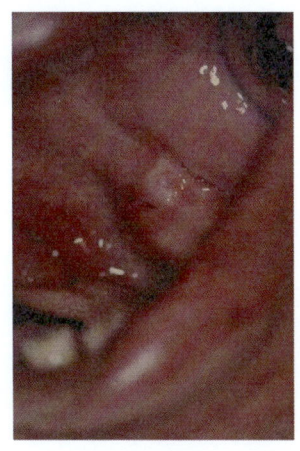

Fig. 139.1.

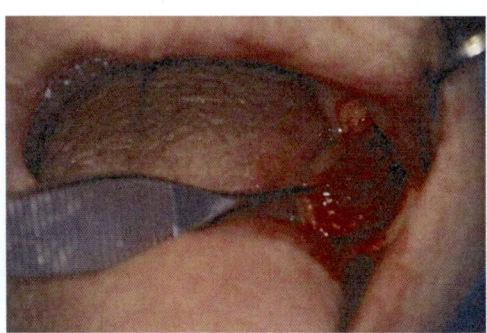

Fig. 139.2.

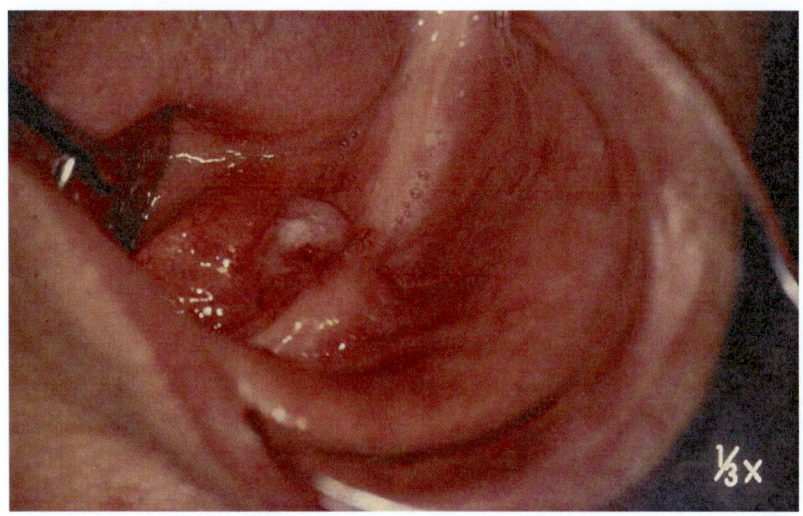

Fig. 139.3.

140. Wegener's granulomatosis

Definition: Systemic necrotizing vasculitis.

Aetiology: Unknown.

Symptoms: Depends on the affected organs. Orally there is pain and bad breath. Bleeding gums.

Clinical features: Usually at 40 to 50 years age. More frequent in men. Granulomatous lesions in the respiratory tract and kidney disease. In 13% of cases there is oral involvement. There is necrosis, ulceration and gingival hyperplasias. Gingiva often have a raspberry-like appearance. Fig.140.1 and Fig.140.2.

Diagnosis: Performed by a biopsy and a histological examination.

Treatment: Refer to a specialist unit.

Differential diagnosis: Tuberculosis. Lymphoma. Leukaemia. Carcinoma.

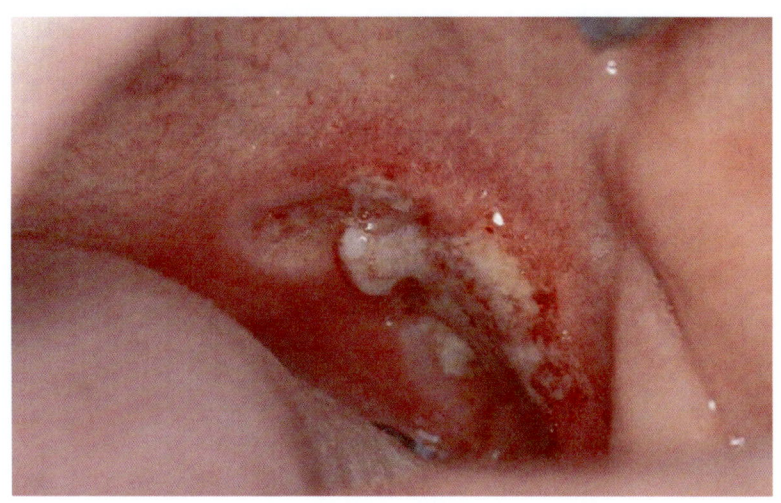

Fig. 140.1.

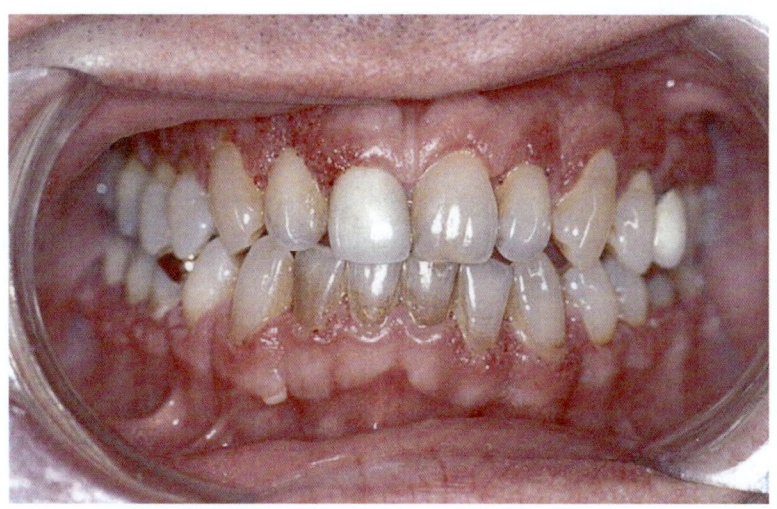

Fig. 140.2.

293

141. Wisdom teeth (pericoronitis)

Definition: Infection around the crown in an emerging wisdom tooth.

Aetiology: Wisdom teeth under eruption often cause the onset of difficulties with infection. This is especially true of the lower jaw wisdom teeth. The wisdom tooth can be mounted abnormally in the jaw. It is often necessary to remove these teeth.
Besides pericoronitis, there may be other reasons for removing a wisdom tooth: Caries, follicular cyst.

Symptoms: Acute pericoronitis causes severe pain, extraoral swelling and trismus. There is sometimes a swollen lymph node, fever and difficulty swallowing.

Clinical features: Trismus, swelling and redness of the skin. Intraorally there is redness and swelling of the wisdom tooth region, and pus from the pocket. Fig.141.1. Pericoronitis can present as an abscessus peritonsillaris or an abscessus cutis, Fig.141.2.

Treatment: Acute infection with pain treated by flushing and with gingiva washing using syringe with 0.1% chlorhexidine and general antibiotics. If there is occlusion directly on the raised mucous membrane flap from the upper jaw wisdom tooth, it can sometimes be beneficial to eliminate this by acute extraction of the maxillary tooth. The definitive treatment is surgical removal of the wisdom tooth.

Differential diagnosis: Tonsillitis. Periodontal abscess.

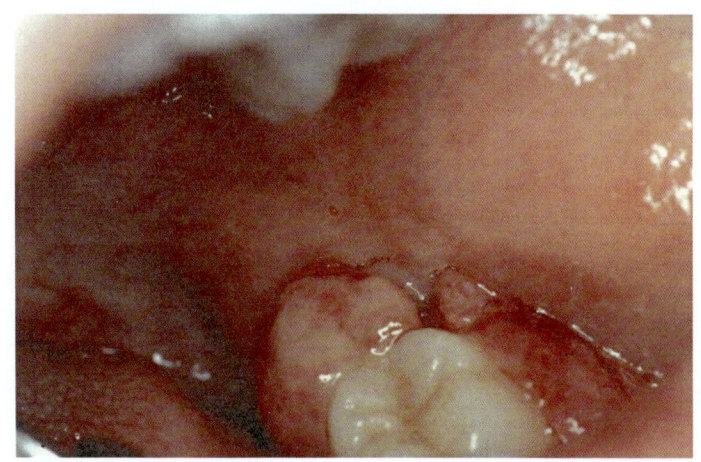

Fig. 141.1.

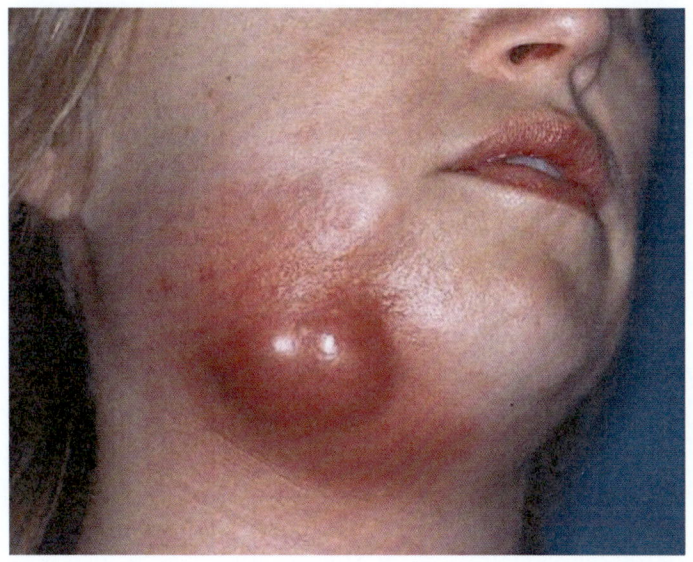

Fig. 141.2.

142. Xerostomia (dry mouth)

Definition: A subjective experience of dryness in the mouth.

Aetiology: Many **medicines** cause dryness in the mouth, such as antidepressants, antihypertensives, antihistamines and sedatives. In addition, some **diseases** cause dry mouth, such as Sjögren's syndrome, Parkinson's disease, depression, diabetes, fever, uremia, anaemia and **radiation** therapy in the head and neck.

Symptoms: The patient has a sense of thirst. He has difficulty eating dry food. Swallowing and speech difficulties. Pain from the mucous membranes. Modified or unpleasant taste and bad breath. **Mb.Sjøgren** is also called sicca syndrome, as there will be dry eyes, dry mouth mucous membrane and rheumatoid arthritis or other connective tissue disease.

Clinical features: Dry mucous membranes Fig.142.1, fissuring and lobulation of the tongue, Fig.142.2, increased incidence of fungus rhagades and dry lips. The saliva is slimy, thick and stringy. Major caries activity, on the tooth neck and on the incisal edges. Fig.142.3.

Diagnosis: Stimulated and unstimulated saliva test. Biopsy of the small salivary glands. Referral to an ophthalmologist and possibly rheumatologist.

Treatment: Examine possibilities for change in medication. Local stimulation of saliva secretion with sugar-free gum and sugar free mints (Xerodent). The patient should also avoid sugary or acidic beverages and foods. Good oral hygiene, frequent dental visits with fluoride treatments are recommended. Rinsing with Flux and Fluoridated gum will reduce the risk of caries.

Differential diagnosis: Sjogren's syndrome. Sequelae after radiotherapy. Medication-induced. Saliva gland pathology.

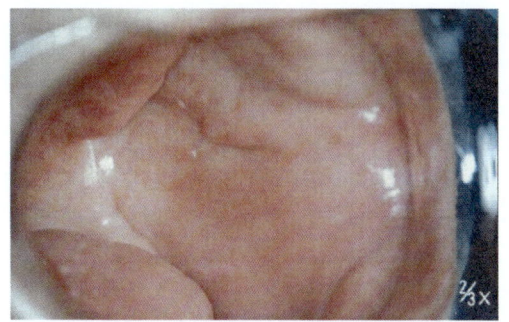

Fig. 142.1.

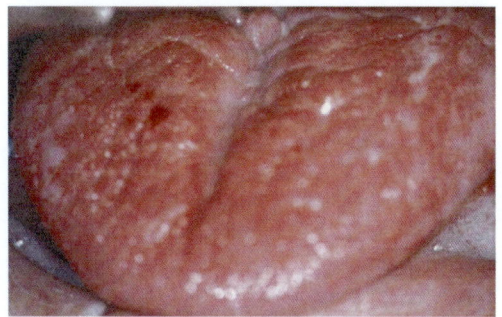

Fig. 142.2.

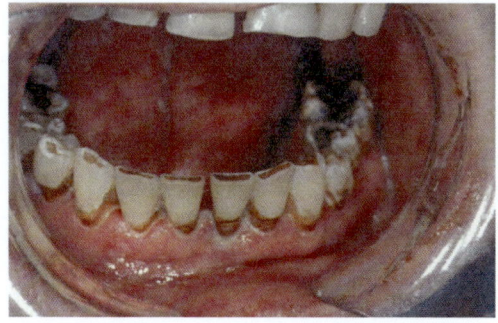

Fig. 142.3.

143. Other specialties

Do it yourself treatment: Some patients have an urge to try to cope themselves with the problems that arise in the teeth and dentures.

Fig.143.1 shows a patient who has fixated loose teeth with plastic padding designed for gutters. On removal, the teeth also came out with individual mites.

Fig.143.2 shows a denture repaired with sewing thread.

Fig.143.3 shows loose periodontal teeth fixed with fishing line.

Fig.143.4 shows an inflammation of the palatine mucous membrane after persistent oro-genital contact (fellatio).

Fig.143.5 shows the result of **Self-mutilation** in a psychiatric patient. The destruction was carried out with the patient's fingernails.

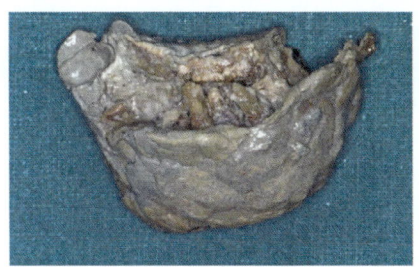 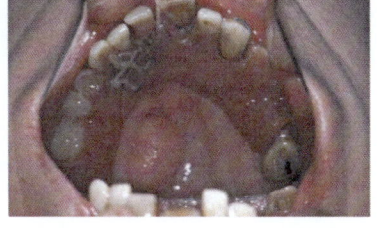

Fig. 143.1.   Fig. 143.2.

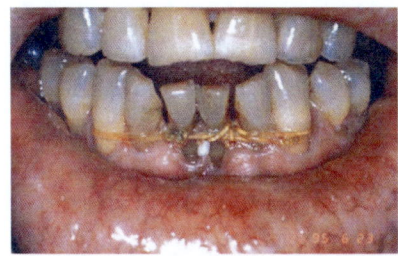 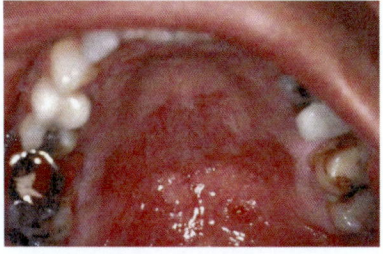

Fig. 143.3.   Fig. 143.4.

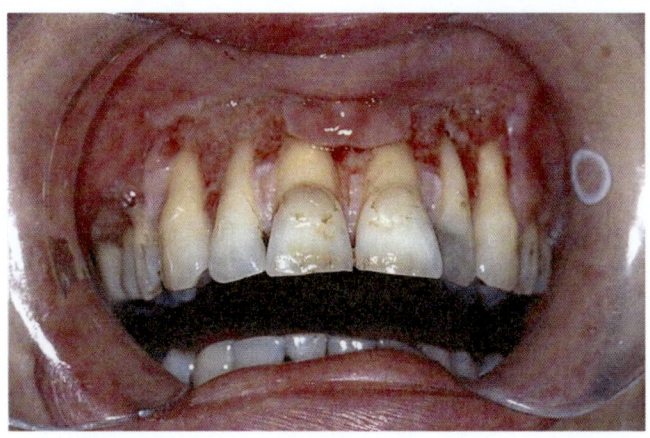

Fig. 143.5.

Electronic literature search

There are a number of medical databases that are of interest to doctors, dentists and other health professionals. We may mention the guidance in MEDLINE in various versions.

MEDLINE is a bibliographic database that is produced by the National Library of Medicine (NLM) in the USA. The database contains references to sources printed in 3,900 biomedicinal journals. Several different hosts - all with their own search engines - provider the database, but it is the same data in all MEDLINE editions. MEDLINE contains references to journal articles written since 1966, and each reference contains information about the title, author, language and keywords (see below) and from 1979 also the author's summary of the article (abstract).

Internet

Today there are several (more than 20) freely available versions of MEDLINE on the Internet. We should highlight two of them: Internet Grateful Med and PubMed. There is the advantage with these Internet editions that they can quickly be updated, so that this is where you should look for if you want to find the latest references in your area of interest. In technical search terms, PubMed is more "advanced" than Internet Grateful Med. Both have the special feature that it is possible to establish links to"related references". This enables you to find other references on the same subject. PubMed also provides the ability to save and subsequently update a search.

Internet Grateful Med has a menu-based search system that makes it easy to use for those not familiar with the searches. In addition, it is possible, besides MEDLINE, also to gain access to a number of other databases of medical interest (e.g. TOXLINE, Health Star and AIDS LINE).

The URL for the two systems is:
http://www.nlm.nih.gov/databases/freemedl.html

Search
Keywords

Information retrieval can either be based on data such as author names, titles, magazines and similar or on the desire to find information within a specific area. To get the full benefits of an item search in Medline, it is important to know the Medical Subject Headings, also called the MeSH system, which is a controlled entry system. The advantage of this is that there is an attempt to ensure consequence and consistency in the choice of tags to the registered references. This means that the use of synonyms and abbreviations will be based on a fixed indexing policy. NLM is the producer of the database and is responsible for developing such guidelines. In PubMed, it is possible to find an explanation and a miniguide on the use of the MeSH system.

Brief guide to the use of Internet Grateful Med

After you have entered the URL
http://www.nlm.nih.gov/databases/freemdl.html
the opening page of both PubMed and Internet Grateful Med comes up on the screen. Click Internet Grateful Med (IGM), and after the introduction page of the IGM will appear on the screen. To the right of the vertical line there is a series of hyperlinks with an introduction and additional information about the system. On the left, under the heading "Select Database to search" a number of databases are specified with MEDLINE on top. At the far left on a blue features, there is an "i", where you can click through to information about the individual databases.

Click the top database MEDLINE, and you will be taken to the IGM's search page. At the top there are a number of action buttons and under the heading "Enter Query Terms" there are three empty boxes where you can enter words to search. You can search by subject, author name or title. In the window the subject form C starting point, but by clicking on the arrow on the right you are shown a drop-down with these three options, which you can then choose.

At the bottom of the page under the heading "Apply Limits" you can limit your search with regard to language study, age etc.. The menus here also have blinds, which you can choose from.

If you want a very precise topic search without non-relevant articles, you need to find and use the current MeSH words. They can be found by using the action button "Find MeSH/Meta Terms". After keying in the word you want, which is closest to the searched topic, click the action button, which will bring a number of possible MeSH words related to the topic. If you click on one of the specified words, you are given a precise definition of the word, and you can find the word's location in the "MeSH tree". When you have chosen the keywords and limited your search, the search itself is started by pressing the action button "Perform Search" either on the bar at the bottom or at the top of the page.

This will display IGM's "Result Screen", where the references found are displayed. The top again shows a number of action buttons, and if you press the "i" to the left you can get further information on them.

Next to each reference there are two fields to the left with the text: "Full Citation" and "Related Articles". Clicking on "Full Citation" makes IGM show the article's abstract, if one exists. If you click on "Related Articles", a number of references in relation to the selected article are displayed. This feature is an extremely useful tool, which is only available in the MEDLINE (PubMed and Grateful Med) database. If desired, you can uncover several subject selections via the "Related Articles". To the left of the references, there is at the top a small square window, where you can select the references which you wish to download.

It is important to know how to use the so-called "Boolean" operators - and ("AND") and or ("OR"). In essence, the boolean operators are used in combined searches. The and operator "AND" describes intersections and the or operator "OR" describes unions. On the search page the default assumption in IGM is that the AND operator is used between the three boxes. You can, by clicking on the far right of the box where it says "add OR", create a new empty box, where another keyword can be written, and then you can search for the union between the two keywords. For a search where you want references concerning oral aspects of, for example, a general disorder, it is recommended to use the MeSH term "oral manifestations" associated with the current conditions of the MeSH term and the operator "AND".

The above is only a very concise and summary guide to searches in IGM. The system also includes a very rich user guide. This is available on IGM's opening page to the right of the triple horizontal line, where you simply click "Users Guide" and possibly also "Training Manual". You will then be guided through the more sophisticated search options in the system.

Diagnostic tree from A to D

A. Colour changes

1. White, abrasion-removable

2. White, not abrasion-removable

3. White and red

4. Red

5. Blue - violet

6. Brown - black

7. Yellow

Candidosis, pseudomembranous

Linea alba	Contact Lesion	Naevus albus spongiosus
Leukoedema	Lichen planus	Friction keratosis
Fordyce spots	Morsicatio	Snus Lesion
Leukoplakia	Smoker's palate	Hairy leukoplakia
Actinic elastosis	Candidosis, plaktype	
(Cheilitis)	LED	

Lingua geographica	Actinic elastosis	LED
Candidosis chronica	Smoker's palate	
Lichen planus	Erythroleukoplakia	

Gingivitis	Lingua Geographica	Anaemia (perniciosa sideropenica)
Stomatitis prothetica	Cheilitis angularis	SLE
Candidosis acuta	haemangioma	Erythroplakia
or chronica	Teleangiektasia	
Glossitis rhombica	Lichen planusmed	
median	Xerostomia/oligosialia	

Amalgam tattoo	Sialocyst	Haemangioma, cavernous
Cystis mucosae oris	Naevus pigmentosus	Mucoepidermoidt carcinoma
Phlebectasia	Giant cell granuloma	Kaposi's sarcoma
Cystis eruptionis	Pregnancy granuloma	Malignant melanoma
Ranula	Pyogenic granuloma	

Ethnic pigmentation	Smokers melanoma	Mb. Addison
Amalgam tattoo	pigmented naevus	Medicine Discoloration
Hairy tongue	Lentigo simplex	Tattoo

Fordyces spots	Salivary Stones	Lipoma
Abscess		

B. Vesiculoerosive and ulcerative lesions

1. Acute

---

2. Chronic

C. Swelling

1. Lower lip

---

2. Upper lip

---

3. Cheek

---

4. Gingiva - alveolar process

Bite wounds	Erythema multiforme	Stomatitis e radiatione
Stomatitis aphthosa	Herpes zoster	Stomatitis medicamentosa
Herpes labialis	Necrotizing	
Primary herpetic	sialometaplasia	
gingivostomatitis	Streptococcal gingivitis	
Secondary herpetic	Leukaemia	
gingivostomatitis		
Ulcer ducubitale	Pemphigus vulgaris	Leukaemia
Lichen, erosive/	Planocellular carcinoma	
ulcerative /ulcerative	Granuloma pyogenicum	
SLE	SARC	
Benign mucous	Neutropenia	
membrane pemfigoid		
Mucocele	Keratoacanthoma	Neurofibroma
Localised fibrous	Mucoepidermoid	Neurilemmoma
hyperplasia	carcinoma	Leiomyoma
Sialocyst	Haemangioma	
Carcinoma	Lipoma	
Localised fibrous	Neurofibroma	Neurilemmoma
hyperplasia	Angio-oedema	Leiomyoma
Adenoma	Melkersson-Rosenthal	
Nasolabial cyst	syndrome	
Localised fibrous	Adenoma	Neurilemmoma
hyperplasia	Haemangioma	Leiomyoma
Lipoma	Neurofibroma	
Mucous membrane cysts	Actinomycosis	
Abscess (periradicular	Hyperplasia gingivae	Metastasis
periodontal)	medicamentosa	Kaposi's sarcoma
Irritation hyperplasia	Fibromatosis gingivae	Haemangioma
(Denture)	Fibroblastic granuloma	Neurofibroma
Pyogenic granuloma	with ossification	Non-Hodgkin's lymphoma
Pregnancy epulis	Peripheral giant	Neurilemmoma
	cell granuloma	

C. Swelling
(Continued)

5. Mouth bottom

6. Tongue

7. Palate

8. Multiple swelling

D. Papillomatous growth

Mucous membrane cysts (Ranula)	Mucoepidermoid carcinoma	Neurofibroma
Salivary Stones	Lipoma	Angio-oedema
Squamous cell carcinoma		Neurilemmoma

Lingua plicata	Mucocele	Amyloidosis
Lingua indentata	Granular cell tumor	Actinomycosis
Papillae foliatae	Lymphangioma	Angio-oedema
Localised fibrous hyperplasia	Haemangioma	Neurilemmoma
Squamous cell carcinoma	Pyogenic granuloma	Leiomyoma
	Mucoepidermoidt carcinoma	

Abscess (periapical, periodontal)	Mucoepidermoidt carcinoma	Necrotizing sialometaplasi
Irritation hyperplasia (Denture)	Polymorphous low-grade adenocarcinoma	Squamous cell carcinoma
Pleomorft adenoma	Kaposi's sarcoma	Non-Hodgkin's lymphoma
Adenoidcystisk carcinoma	Fibroma	Neurilemmom
		Leiomyoma

Kaposi's sarcoma	Focal epithelial hyperplasia	Angio-oedema
Neurofibromatosis	Amyloidosis	

Hairy tongue	Non-homogeneous (verrucous)	Condyloma acuminatum
Papilloma		Focal epithelial hyperplasia
Stomatitis prothetica	Squamous cell carcinoma	
Verruca vulgaris	Verrucous carcinoma	